Tantra

–

Discovering the Power
of
Pre-Orgasmic Sex

Yogani

From The AYP Enlightenment Series

AYP Publishing

For ordering information go to:

www.advancedyogapractices.com

Library of Congress Control Number: 2006923698

Published simultaneously in:

Nashville, Tennessee, U.S.A.
and
London, England, U.K.

This title is also available in eBook format – ISBN 0-9764655-9-0
(For Adobe Reader)

ISBN 0-9764655-8-2 (Paperback)

"At the start of sexual union, keep attention on the fire *in the beginning*, and, so continuing, avoid the embers in the end."

Vigyan Bhairava (4,000 year-old scripture)
Zen Flesh, Zen Bones – Transcribed by Paul Reps

Introduction

The ancient field of *Tantra* is so broad that it defies description. Not only does it include all of the practices contained in the traditional systems of Yoga; it also contains practices that, at times, have challenged the established codes and standards of society. The sexual practices of tantra fall under this controversial category.

Human sexuality has an essential role to play in the conduct of practices aimed at accelerating the natural process of human spiritual transformation.

This book is a common-sense guide on how to utilize our sexuality to complement a full-scope system of yoga practices. Practical techniques are provided which enable both couples and solo practitioners to use the sexual response to cultivate ecstatic energy to its highest levels of spiritual manifestation in support of the journey to enlightenment.

The Advanced Yoga Practices Enlightenment Series is an endeavor to present the most effective methods of spiritual practice in a series of easy-to-read books that anyone can use to gain practical results immediately and over the long term. For centuries, these powerful practices have been taught in secret, mainly in an effort to preserve them. Now we find ourselves in the *information age*, and able to preserve knowledge for present and future generations like never before. The question remains:

"How far can we go in effectively transmitting spiritual methods in writing?"

Since its beginnings in 2003, the writings of *Advanced Yoga Practices* have been an experiment to see just how much can be conveyed, with much more detail included on practices than in the spiritual writings of the past. Can books provide us the specific means necessary to tread the path to enlightenment, or do we have to surrender at the feet of a *guru* to find our salvation? Well, clearly we must surrender to something, even if it is to our own innate potential to live a freer and happier life. If we are able to do that, and maintain a daily practice, then books like this one can come alive and instruct us in the ways of human spiritual transformation. If the reader is ready and the book is worthy, amazing things can happen.

While one person's name is given as the author of this book, it is actually a distillation of the efforts of thousands of practitioners over thousands of years. This is one person's attempt to simplify and make practical the spiritual methods that many have demonstrated throughout history. All who have gone before have my deepest gratitude, as do the many I am privileged to be in touch with in the present who continue to practice with dedication and good results.

I hope you will find this book to be a useful resource as you travel along your chosen path.

Practice wisely, and enjoy!

Table of Contents

Chapter 1 – Tantra, Sex and Spirituality

Sex has an essential role to play in the process of human spiritual transformation. In these times, the word "tantra" has become synonymous with "spiritual sex." But tantra is far more than that. It may well be the broadest system of spiritual practices in the world, encompassing all of yoga, and then some, leaving literally nothing out in terms of the many means that can be applied to accelerate our spiritual progress. So, in that sense, tantra sometimes gets a "bad rap," because, in addition to meditation, pranayama (breathing techniques), postures and numerous other aspects of practice, it also includes sexual practices. And we humans, being the sexually fixated beings that we are, say, "Tantra is about sex!" The analysis of tantra usually proceeds accordingly, along sexual lines, for better or for worse.

And so too shall we follow the sexual angle here in discussing tantra, not because the other practices are not important (they are very important and are covered fully in the other AYP writings), but because sex has a unique role to play in spiritual practices and in our transformation to higher states of consciousness. To ignore this is to ignore an essential part of our path and our potential to enjoy growing fulfillment and happiness. So, in this book, we will give sex its due. Then, along the way, we show the connection between tantric sexual principles and the other traditional aspects of yoga.

Contrary to long-entrenched beliefs, sex is not the enemy of spiritual progress. In truth, sex can be a powerful ally, if understood for what it is and harnessed in an intelligent way. There are a variety of means for accomplishing this, with each being suited to the personal inclinations of particular kinds of spiritual practitioners. In every case the underlying principle is the same – the pre-orgasmic cultivation of sexual energy toward an increasing manifestation of our inherent ecstatic nature over the long term. Once we have experienced this, even a little, then a whole new permanent inner world will begin to open to us. This is in contrast to the transient nature of reproductive sex.

It is funny, you know, how a perception has crystallized as tantra has crept toward the mainstream of our modern society. The common perception for most these days is that tantra is about sex – better sex, more ecstatic sex, more *spiritual sex*. So the call of tantra has become, "Sex, sex, sex!" Do we have one-track minds, or what? It is natural enough. For most of us, the peak experience of our life is found in the sex act, particularly in the overwhelming pleasure of orgasm. So it is no surprise that we are a culture obsessed with sex – usually for it, sometimes against it, and always in awe of it. We all know that sex somehow connects us with a greater dimension of what we are. It is a fact that sex binds us together in love, family and, ultimately, our spiritual life. So, of course we are obsessed with sex. It lies at the root of everything we are. It defines us. A deep desire we all have is to merge permanently with the ecstasy contained in this thing called "sex."

To unravel the ultimate mystery of sex, we will be wise to take a broad view of it. This is where tantra comes in.

What if I told you that tantra is mainly about meditation, pranayama (breathing techniques), and other *sitting practices* that we do like clockwork on a daily basis? It is true that tantra is mainly about these things. Yes, tantra is about sex too, and we must face up to it if we wish to progress on our path. Enlightenment is not possible if our sexuality is not brought into the process of yoga – the process of union between our inner divine self and the outer world. In cultivating our nervous system toward that, the role of sexual energy must be addressed.

Tantra means "woven together," or "two fullnesses as one." It means the same thing as yoga really – *union*, with intimacy added. Tantra recognizes from the start that there are two poles to be ecstatically merged for enlightenment to occur – father heaven and mother earth, masculine and feminine energies, shiva and shakti, yin and yang –

and that these two poles are contained in us, in our nervous system. This has practical implications in our daily life.

Tantra is the broadest of all the yoga systems that approach life as two realities to be joined in the human nervous system. Included within tantra are mantra yoga, kriya yoga, kundalini yoga, hatha yoga, ashtanga (eight-limbed) yoga, and others. The practices contained in these traditional yoga systems comprise what is called the *right-handed* side of tantra. Then there is the *left-handed* side of tantra yoga, which is concerned with infusing pure bliss consciousness into the indulgences of sensual life in the material world. The left-handed side is not opposed to sensual indulgences. In fact, it takes advantage of them for spiritual purposes. The left-handed side is sort of the underbelly of yoga, the part that upstanding citizens are supposed to stay away from. That is the traditional view anyway. That was before the *hip generation* got a hold of tantra. Now it is respectable to practice left-handed tantra. At least in the West it is. Maybe Westerners don't have anything to lose, being so immersed in material living to begin with. Why not bring the spiritual side into our material living? Let's have our cake and eat it too. It's got left-handed tantra written all over it.

So, in this book, we will take a closer look at left-handed tantra as it pertains to sexual methods.

What we will find is connections with principles and practices we cover in the other AYP writings. In those writings, we fully discuss *kundalini* – the vast latent energy inherent in our sexual biology, which is systematically awakened and managed with advanced yoga practices. These practices stimulate ecstatic sexual energy upward to permeate our nervous system on a full-time basis, and are incorporated into our twice-daily routine of sitting practices, which has deep meditation and spinal breathing pranayama at its core. The additional practices aimed at expanding the role of our sexual energy for spiritual transformation are in the category of *asanas, mudras and bandhas*.

All of these sitting practices are operating from the root (perineum) on up. In reviewing tantric sexual methods, we are going to go below the root, so to speak. It is necessary. For if we do not get a handle on the huge flows of prana (life force) involved in the sex act, we may find that we are limited in what we can accomplish spiritually in our nervous system. This does not mean we have to entertain the dreaded "C" word – *celibacy*. It does mean we will consider some intelligent methods to bring our sexual activities more in line with our spiritual aspirations. In fact, you may be surprised to find that intelligent spiritual sex can be far more enjoyable than the run-of-the-mill kind of sex which is sometimes characterized by the phrase, "Wham, bam, thank you Ma'am."

How will we know if we are ready for tantric sexual techniques? It is easy enough. We will want to do something *regenerative* with our sex life. It will become important to us. The more we want it the better it will be. This desire is called *bhakti*. The level of bhakti in us is easy to feel, and easy for others to notice as well. It comes as the nervous system purifies itself as a result of our yoga practices. It is a kind of magnetism that rises calling us toward more. It takes a strong call to get us into a new spiritually oriented mode of sexual activity, because we have to do something radical. It takes a radical desire to undertake tantric sex. We are embarking on a journey to alter the course of a mighty river. In tantric sex, we are learning to engage in sex for the purpose of cultivating sexual energy upward, and putting our deeply ingrained obsession for orgasm second. Spiritual cultivation of sexual energy first, orgasm second – a big shift in our aspirations. If our desire is strong, we will be able to expand our sexual functioning to a cultivating mode, just as we train our arousal brought up with certain sitting practices to a much higher functioning over time. It is like that in tantric sex – a gradual training over a long period of time. Tantric sex is not an overnight accomplishment. It is an evolution over time – over many months and years. As our bhakti strengthens it will happen, because it must to fulfill our journey to enlightenment.

The sexual journey through yoga will not be the same for everyone. It will be as different for each of us as our sexual inclinations are.

For those who are light to moderate in their sex life, there is not a great necessity to introduce yogic methods into sexual relations, though learning tantric sex certainly will enhance lovemaking, and the rest of our yoga practices as well. Occasional sex is not much of a deterrent to enlightenment. The traditional methods of yoga (right-handed tantra) discussed in the over all AYP writings will be more than enough to get the job done.

For those who are very active in sex, it is a different story. Though the storehouse of prana (life force) in the pelvis is huge, there is a limit to how much one can expel and still be spiritually vibrant. This is especially true for men, where large quantities of prana are released during orgasm with the ejaculation of semen. It is somewhat true for women also, but not to the same degree. It is the man who holds the keys to tantric sex, for it is he who experiences the greatest loss of prana during orgasm. Because of this, it is also he who determines the duration of the sexual joining and, therefore, the extent of cultivation of sexual energy that can occur during lovemaking. While a woman may be filled with bhakti/desire to bring sexual energy higher and higher in herself and her partner, it is the man's bhakti that will determine to what extent this can be accomplished in sexual union. So the roles of a man and woman in tantric sex are somewhat different. Yet, in another way, their roles are the same. For tantric sex to occur, both the man and the woman must be involved in the intelligent management of the man's ejaculation. This is true in the beginning stages of learning tantric sex, and remains true for some time.

In time, and with practice, the man becomes the master of his semen and is no longer dependent on help from his partner to control his ejaculation. When this level of proficiency has been reached, both partners are free to cultivate sexual energy pre-orgasmically virtually indefinitely. We have all seen Asian visual art of tantric lovers in union playing musical instruments, reading poetry, meditating, or joined in long loving conversation. This is not usually what we think of in the West as sex, or even tantric sex. Nevertheless, this is what real tantric sex is – long pre-orgasmic cultivation of sexual energy in lovemaking.

It is important to mention a couple of things.

First, tantric sex does not make a good end in itself. It does not stand alone as yoga practice. By itself, tantric sex is a weak practice for globally purifying and opening the nervous system. It won't work. Deep meditation and spinal breathing pranayama are the primary tools for this. Once some purification is coming up, asanas, mudras, bandhas and kumbhaka (breath suspension) are very useful for stimulating sexual energy upward. This leads to a rise of *ecstatic conductivity* in the *sushumna* (the spinal nerve running from the bottom of the pelvis up to the brain) and throughout the tens of thousands of nerves fanning out from the spine to every part of the body. Tantric sex can play a role in this, especially for sexually active yogis and yoginis (a *yogi* is a male practitioner of yoga, and a *yogini* is a female practitioner). Tantric sex is not something we do to get ourselves to be more sexually active. It is something we can do to improve our yoga if we are already sexually active. So, this discussion is not for the purpose of calling everyone to have more sex in a tantric mode. If you are light to moderate in sex and happy in your yoga practices, you are in very good shape. Don't dive into sexual escapades for the sake of what you are reading here. This book on tantric sex is for people who are sexually active already and are seeking ways to bring their sexual activity into the overall spectrum of their yoga practice.

Second, it may seem like a bad idea to some that we are leaving orgasm somewhat on the back shelf while we develop the ability to cultivate sexual energy endlessly upward. It might seem like we are throwing the baby out with the bath water here. After all, orgasm is the deepest pleasure we have known in our life. This is a normal and valid concern, and we are right to ask, "What about orgasm? What happens to it?"

These writings are not anti-orgasm. In fact, the path recommended in the AYP writings is a path of pleasure, a path of ecstasy. Orgasm is an ecstatic response in the body that is elicited by a particular type of stimulation – sexual stimulation that is biologically oriented toward reproduction. The condition in the nervous system that we call *enlightenment* is also an ecstatic response in the body that is elicited by a particular type of stimulation – stimulation by yoga practices that is biologically oriented toward the birth of our awareness in unending pure bliss consciousness and divine ecstasy.

Is enlightenment at the expense of orgasm? No, enlightenment is a flowering of orgasm, an expansion of orgasm into endless full bloom in the whole body.

The great 19th century Indian sage, Ramakrishna, said that divine ecstasy is like innumerable yonis (female sex organs) in continual orgasm in every atom and pore of our body.

So, while in the beginning it might seem like we are putting something important on the back shelf, what we are really doing is gradually expanding our orgasmic response into the cosmic realms through our purifying and opening nervous system. There we find ecstasy to be unbounded in magnitude and duration. It is only a matter of cultivating our nervous system to reveal what is already there inside us.

It is through our bhakti/desire that all this is accomplished. Each day we choose our path anew.

Okay, let's get into the specifics of the practices of tantric sex.

Chapter 2 – Tantric Sexual Practices

The essential principle involved in all the methods of tantric sexual practices is the pre-orgasmic cultivation of sexual energy. This can be done with a partner, alone in solo sexual practice, and in traditional sitting yoga practices. We will look at all of these in the course of our discussion here. But before any of that, something *a priori* (before the fact) is needed. That something is desire. The power of sexual instinct is so powerful that a considerable desire for something more (also called *bhakti*) must be there before we will find much progress with tantric sexual methods.

The Power of Intention

It is common knowledge that if we want to be successful at something, at anything, we must desire it continuously, and be willing to act to fulfill that desire every day. Intention is at the heart of our doing. Think of the most successful people you know. Isn't this what they have in common? If we look at their lives, we see that they have worked long and hard to achieve excellence in their chosen field. Behind that, an insatiable desire to succeed in their efforts kept them driving forward, overcoming obstacles, working for years toward their objective. It is like that in tantra, which is working toward an awakening and a divine union within us.

Jesus said, "Blessed are those who hunger and thirst after righteousness, for they shall be filled." He also said, "Seek and you will find. Knock and the door will open to you."

This is the magic formula – desire toward a goal, which spawns action toward that goal. Continuous desire is the fuel. Daily action is the fire. The word *continuous* is important, as is the word *goal*. Without these two operative functions, desires are scattered, actions are unfocused, and not much happens. With them, anything is achievable.

If we cultivate our desire to become continuously focused on a particular goal, such as the achievement of divine union via tantric means, we are cultivating a special kind of desire. It is called *devotion*. Devotion is the continuous flow of desire toward an object or goal. We are all familiar with the concept of devotion. It is how we explain the success of great achievers: "Oh, she is so devoted to her work." Or of great mystics: "Oh, she is so devoted to God." It is no coincidence that devotion and greatness are found in the same place. The first invariably leads to the second. The second cannot happen without the first.

Whatever your concept of sexual fulfillment or enlightenment may be, whatever tradition or creed you hail from, whatever inspires you in the direction of spiritual unfoldment, cultivate that. It is the engine of all practice. It is what enables us to sustain daily spiritual practice for as long as it takes. As we practice, our divine experience grows, and, with that, devotion grows. Increased devotion intensifies our commitment to practice, and more dedicated practice yields more divine experience which in turn increases devotion further. This is how it progresses – devotion yielding practice ... yielding divine experience ... yielding more devotion ... and so on. Devotion sustained at a fever pitch by every means possible is the spiritual aspirant's best friend. It is not always an easy life being constantly consumed by spiritual *hunger and thirst*, but it puts us on the royal road to enlightenment. Intense devotion to transforming our lives through yoga practices and tantric methods assures that what must be done will be done.

The Holdback Technique – A Stairway to Heaven

What is perfect lovemaking? Is there such a thing? It is like asking, "What is enlightenment?" Maybe they are the same thing. Whatever they may be in the end, we have to begin from where we are. There is a process we can undertake, a journey. If we believe there is something more, we can begin from where we are and move forward. It takes a continuous desire to make the journey.

There are so many factors in sexual relations. Compatibility is a big one. Do we get along? Are we good in bed together? There are many nuances of personal preference and style that we are seeking to match up to our liking. Am I attractive? Is he/she attractive? Is the flirting right? Is the foreplay good? Is the place of lovemaking suitable – the bedroom, the basement, the kitchen table?

Here, we will not focus much on these things. They are important for sure. But what we want to focus on here is the act itself. Specifically, how prana (our life force expressing as sexual energy) is affected during sexual stimulation, and what we can do to bring that stimulation into the realm of yoga practice. Obviously, an important part of this is answering the question, "What do I want from sex?" If the answer is, "Something more than genital orgasm," then we are ready to begin experimenting with tantric sexual methods.

The methods are pretty simple. It is about managing sexual stimulation and orgasm. And it is about male plumbing (piping). Very mundane stuff when you think about it. But we bring so much baggage to the bed with us, you know – our obsessions about sex. And that can make it a bit complicated. But it doesn't have to be complicated.

We have obsessions, strong emotional reactions relating to sex. Let's remind ourselves that we are coming to the bed for a higher purpose in lovemaking, and let's use bhakti/desire to direct our sexual obsessions to that. A little bhakti can go a long way.

An important part of this higher purpose is to remember that tantric sex is about our partner's needs. If both partners take this to heart, then there will be great success in tantric sex, or any sex, or any relationship. It is like a Buddhist koan, an unsolvable riddle. If both partners are looking to serve the other, who is being served? If personal need has been transcended, whose need is being filled?

Of course, serving our partner 100% is an ideal, a goal to be gradually fulfilled over a long time. Let your attention come to it easily from time to time as you are making love. It will make a difference. If you are coming to tantric sex sincerely (you probably had this in mind already), then it is about honoring and filling your partner with divine ecstasy. So, take this as a confirmation of what you already instinctively know. Tantric sex is about your partner. Of course, both partners will not always have equal concern for each other. That is okay. Giving does not require a response in kind. Lovemaking is not a business transaction. Lovemaking is making "love." We make love by giving, by doing for someone other than ourselves, not expecting a return for it. This is what love is. It is not necessarily about making a lifetime commitment. It is not about the future or the past. It is just about serving in this very moment.

Sometimes making love means saying, "no." Loving is not rolling over for every desire our partner may have, particularly a desire that is destructive. Under these circumstances, saying, "no" is loving too. Love isn't a pushover. Love is wise. Love is strong. Love radiates peace and light to all of life. This is an important part of what we want to cultivate in tantric sex. It will happen naturally as we progress.

So, these are the foundation blocks:

First, understanding that tantric sex is about cultivating sexual energy upward pre-orgasmically in our nervous system. Second, that sitting yoga practices (meditation, pranayama, etc.) discussed in other AYP writings can provide prerequisite purification in our nervous system. Third, that we are looking for more than genital orgasm. And fourth, that we are there for our partner.

Now let's talk about the holdback method.

We will refer to the male organ as the *lingam* and the female organ as the *yoni*. These are the traditional Sanskrit names used in tantra for the masculine and feminine organs of regeneration, covering the full scope of ecstatic union from the physical to the highest spiritual.

The holdback method is most easily done with the man on top and the woman on the bottom. It can be done in other positions also once the partners become familiar with the principles. It is the most difficult to do with the woman on top, as will become evident.

When a man and woman are in lovemaking, the holdback method involves just what it says – holding back. It is done by the man. It is done before his orgasm, preferably not too close to his orgasm. The idea is not to get to the edge of orgasm and then hold back. It can be too late then, and then the man is out of business until next time. No doubt it will happen that way sometimes, and that is okay. We will discuss another method in the next section to help with that. For now, let's continue with the holdback method.

Intercourse is simulative stroking, yes? This is the natural way it goes until the man has orgasm. Maybe the woman has orgasm first, maybe not. But when the man has orgasm it is over, at least for a while. He may come back soon in a semi-recovered state to try and satisfy his lover, and then maybe lose more semen. She may find some satisfaction, but he has paid a high price, energy-wise. If this goes on daily for a long time, the man's progress in yoga practices will suffer. The woman's progress in yoga won't be helped much either. If it happens only once a week, or less often, it is not such a big deal. But even those who have sex only occasionally can find their yoga progress improved by knowing the methods of tantric sex.

Mastery of the holdback method changes the dynamic of this old style of orgasmic sex, introducing a new dynamic of pre-orgasmic sex with many benefits.

In the holdback method, the lingam enters the yoni for a number of strokes and then pulls out and lingers around the opening of the yoni. How many strokes is up to the man, but well short of orgasm is recommended. This is supposed to be a long lovemaking, so holding back sooner rather than later is best in the beginning, as this is when the staying power will be least in most men. A few things are going on when the lingam is in holdback mode. First, the staying power of the man in front of orgasm is being strengthened, recharging to a higher level of staying power than before the previous entry into the yoni. Second, the woman is in anticipation, and this is sexually exciting for her. She does not know when the lingam is coming back into her, and this anticipation will increase her arousal. To add to the woman's anticipation and excitement, the man may do a little teasing with the tip of his lingam, without risking his own orgasm. He may enter the yoni just a little bit and then pull back out. Or he may not touch the yoni at all with his lingam, and then all of a sudden when she least expects it ... Well, use your imagination. An accomplished tantric man won't use the same pattern of stroking and lingering twice in a row. There are lots of ways to play the game.

Everyone will play the game a little differently. That is fine. It is the principles of practice we are after that tap into the natural ability of the nervous system to bring ecstatic energy ever higher in the body.

The important thing in using the holdback method is for the man to pull out in time and give himself adequate time to recharge and increase his staying power. In the beginning this means relaxing outside the yoni for a while and not rushing back in as soon as the lingam has been out for a few seconds. In the beginning, it is all about building up staying power in the man, and this is done by stroking inside pre-orgasmically and stopping outside, over and over again. This practice can immediately level the playing field between the man and woman in sexual relations.

Everyone knows that the woman is superior to the man in the sex act, and in other things as well. Nature has built her to be biologically superior in sexual relations. The survival of the human race depends on it. She will have the semen no matter what. She does not even have to try. Her beauty calls the semen from the man on sight. Her curves, her lips, her eyes, all call the semen out.

Hundreds of years ago the great reviver of yoga in India, Shankara, is reported to have said, "Even the greatest yogi cannot gaze into the eyes of a beautiful woman without having his seed jump."

With knowledge of the holdback method we can balance sexual relations to the benefit of both the man and the woman. Over time, the man's staying power becomes very great, even from the beginning of a lovemaking session. A change occurs gradually in his sexual biology as a result of using the holdback method. This brings freedom to both partners in lovemaking, and solves the challenge of sex that Shankara pointed out.

As we progress with the holdback method we discover that we are on a new path in our sexual relations. It involves longer sex, which is a boon to both the man and the woman. But with the holdback method we get much more than length. We get height, which is the greatest payoff.

What do we mean by height? As the man goes through the cycles of stroking and holding back, a stairway of rising ecstasy is being climbed. Of course, the woman is not inert in this process. She is active every step of the way – coaxing her man when he is in her, and becoming more aroused with anticipation each time he lingers near her entrance. There is stimulation, and then pause, more stimulation and then pause, and so on. With each cycle the pleasure rises. The essences of love, sexual energy, rise to permeate the bodies of the two in lovemaking. Together they go up the stairs of ecstasy being created by the repeating cycles of stimulation and pauses. It is a stairway to heaven.

The holdback method has also been called the *valley orgasm* method. The partners go up the side of the mountain of stimulation toward genital orgasm. Then they pause before they get there and slowly dip into a valley of pleasure higher than where they started. Then they go up with stimulation toward genital orgasm again, stopping before they get there, and dip back into a valley of pleasure again, this one higher than the first. And then they do it again, and again, and again. The mountains and valleys get higher and higher. In the end, the lovers are permeated with sexual essences, gone into a bliss state akin to deep meditation.

This is how sexual relations are turned into yoga practice.

That is the holdback method. This is not a practice you are supposed to do for so many minutes twice a day. It is for doing in your normal love life, whatever that may be. Maybe sex is not of much interest to you. Then you won't need any of this. It is here for those who need it, and not here to promote more sex. What we want to promote is more yoga practices. Tantric sex is only one aspect of a large array of tools we have in AYP to purify and open our nervous system to higher experiences of the divine within us.

Next we will talk about getting a better handle on male orgasm. It is not likely that knowing the holdback method alone will be enough for all men to stay in front of orgasm right from the beginning, even with a great desire to do it. It is not an easy thing to master. It takes some special self-training.

Transforming Male Orgasm

The holdback method is pretty straightforward. There is only one catch to it. Many men have little or no control over their orgasm. And in the heat of the moment they don't want any control. The semen wants to go, and that is it. Sex is a mad dash for that, and everything else tends to fall by the wayside.

So, how do we get around this? The key is in altering the habit of the inner neurology of orgasm. We do this by giving the male neurology a familiarity with a different way of traveling the road of stimulation. In doing so, we find a different experience of pleasure, and the experience of divine ecstasy coming up through the nervous system. In time, divine ecstasy becomes more charming than the jerking and lurching of genital orgasm, and we become motivated to spend more time in the habit of pre-orgasmic stimulation. We then have the choice –

pre-orgasmic tantric sex or genital orgasm. Maybe in a single session we'd like to have both, beginning with a long session of the former and finally ending with the latter. Once in a while, why not? That is having the cake and eating it too. Of course, do that too often (like more than every week or two) and the cake will be eating up your yoga.

In principle, the holdback method alone can provide the necessary training for the man. We will talk about the woman's evolving role in tantric sex in the next section. She is very important, obviously. But first, we have to deliver her a motivated tantric man. Without that, there won't be much tantric sex going on. That is why we are focusing on the man first.

Is the holdback method enough for training the man's orgasmic response? Maybe for some it is, especially if they are experienced and have been working seriously on lasting before orgasm already. But for many, the holdback method will not be enough.

We will now talk about blocking male ejaculation. It is an ancient tantric method with a long history of success. It is simple enough to do.

When orgasm is about to come on, the man puts one or two fingers (usually index and/or middle finger) at the perineum, the area between the anus and the root of the lingam, presses inward and forward against the back of the pubic bone, and blocks the urethra channel that the semen is about to come through. The orgasm still occurs, but the semen is blocked from leaving the body. If the man lets go too soon, the semen can still escape. If he holds the block for a minute or two and then let's go, the semen will be reabsorbed and none will escape.

Blocking can be done by reaching to the perineum from either the front or the back. In tantric lovemaking with a partner, the man can reach from the back and block his ejaculation if he has slipped and gone too far with stimulation. He still has orgasm and will be done with sex for a while, but he has blocked the loss of semen from his orgasm.

Beyond the mechanics of stopping the exit of semen from the body, the blocking method has several other aspects related to training the orgasmic response of the man.

First, having an orgasm with the ejaculation blocked is initially not nearly as pleasurable as having one with a free flow of semen. If a man's bhakti brings him to engage in blocking most of his ejaculations, then there will also be a gradual shift in his motivation from wanting to go to orgasm to wanting to stay in front of it. So, blocking, besides stopping semen from leaving, provides an incentive for a man to stay in front of orgasm. Why go there if it is going to be less pleasurable than continuing in pre-orgasmic sex and climbing that stairway to heaven with our lover?

Second, given what has just been said, blocking is not something that will be needed forever. It is a voluntary, temporary measure, like having training wheels on a bicycle. Aren't you glad to hear that? Bicycles with training wheels are not much fun. We want to get them off as soon as possible so we can ride free. So we have an additional incentive to train our orgasmic response and reduce our reliance on the training wheels. Once we learn to stay in pre-orgasmic in sex for long periods, we won't need blocking very often. By the time we get to that stage, having genital orgasm may be part of sex only after an hour or two in union, or maybe we will forget about it completely.

Forget about orgasm? Yes, the experiences in long tantric sex can become so profound that we can forget about orgasm completely. Hard to believe, but it is true. Tantric sex can be that good. And it is good yoga practice too! Over time, the importance of the genital orgasm will fade to the background. We can still have it if we want it, but it will become less attractive as our divine ecstasy expands beyond it. Sex will still be good, but in a different way. Sex will become an expression of our overall rising enlightenment, rather than the obsessive needful thing it has been in the past.

Now we should talk about male masturbation.

It was mentioned that blocking can be done from the front or the back. If a man is masturbating, the blocking can come in from the front. Given the fact that the total semen expelled in masturbation in the lifetime of an average man exceeds the amount expelled in lovemaking many-fold, we should really talk about it.

Masturbation is the greatest expeller of semen for many men. Masturbation also happens to be an advantageous time to be training the male orgasm. It is a good time to practice the equivalent of the holdback method, holding back before orgasm over and over again, and permanently building the staying power to a high level. It is also a good time to practice blocking when orgasm comes. So, all the elements are there. Stimulation, pauses, and blocking as necessary. Only the partner is missing. Interestingly, this is not far from what we are doing with the traditional methods of mudras, bandhas and other yoga practices – stimulating our pre-orgasmic sexual energy systematically up through our nervous system.

So, is tantric masturbation a kind of yoga practice? Yes, it can be as long as it remains pre-orgasmic. It is also an ideal self-training ground for a man to prepare for tantric sex with a partner.

None of this is to promote excessive sexual activity, or more masturbation than is already going on. It is just to add an awareness of tantric methods that can be incorporated into what we are already doing in our sex life. If we do so intelligently, dramatic changes in our experience of sex can be achieved, and our overall yoga practices will be enhanced significantly.

The Woman as Divine Goddess

Now that we have given the man the primary tools that will enable him to work toward having a strong role in tantric sexual relations, let's talk about the role of the woman.

The woman is everything in tantric sex, and in all of life. She is the *divine goddess*. Everything we see and everything we do is born of the divine feminine. That is why, in this world, she is called *Mother Nature*. It is the divine feminine that attracts the masculine seed of pure bliss consciousness and manifests all. The cosmos and everything in it is born from Her.

When a man and woman engage in sexual relations, it is a microcosm of this great divine process. In tantric sex involving accomplished partners, it begins as a microcosm and rises toward the cosmic joining of the masculine seed and feminine womb. This joining occurs in both the man and the woman. This expanding ecstatic event fulfills itself inside each of the partners as they engage in tantric sex together, and also as each does their sitting yoga practices in their meditation room. This joining of masculine and feminine energies occurs in many ways. It threads its way through all of our yoga practices – deep meditation, spinal breathing pranayama and so on. Everything in yoga is about this spiritual joining that occurs on every level in the nervous system.

So, when a man and woman come together in tantric sex, this is the beginning of something much bigger in both of them, reaching far beyond the bodies present on the bed. The man's role is seed, whether he is giving it physically or not. If he does not give it physically, it is cultivated up in both partners spiritually.

The woman's role is divine goddess, the flower garden of ecstatic bliss. She calls the seed from the man. If it does not come physically, it comes up and fertilizes from within both partners spiritually. The more she calls, the more the fertilizing will happen. If not physically, then spiritually. She is the inspiration of both physical and spiritual fertilization. This is the essence of the woman's role in tantric sex. She is the temptress of the physical seed, and the temptress of the spiritual seed. If the physical seed does not come, the spiritual seed will. Her lovely divine bliss and waves of beauty will bring the seed out. If the man is able to hold the physical seed back, then the spiritual seed rises in both the man and the woman, and this is the internal joining of masculine and feminine energies in both tantric partners.

Tantric sex is about that – about stimulating the internal divine union in both partners. It is the same purpose that is found in all yoga practices. If both partners in tantric sex have been doing yoga practices daily on their own, then there will be much purification in their nervous systems already, and tantric sex will be much more effective. The sexual essences will rise and penetrate their nervous systems deeply, and the experience will be like the deepest meditation, rich in pure silence, ecstatic bliss and overflowing with love. This will carry over into daily activity and the regular routine of spiritual practices. So tantric sex can have this very positive and profound effect in life. For people who are sexually active, this is the beautiful silver lining in the dark cloud that sex can sometimes hang over spiritual life.

It takes discipline to get to such a wonderful stage of lovemaking. We talked about the challenges the man faces in learning to become the master of his semen, and what methods he can use. What can the woman do to help this evolution toward tantric sexual relations?

Obviously, her first responsibility is to understand the process of transformation to tantric sexual relations – understanding that it involves cultivating a change in the man's orgasmic response, and that this is not an overnight change. Her partner may not understand this at the start. She has the ability to educate him. Before a divine goddess will be able to engage in tantric sexual relations she may find herself becoming a teacher, a tantric priestess, if you will. This can be very helpful to a man trying to understand his sexuality. But she can only do so much, for it is he who must take up the challenge. A tantric woman cannot do the holdback method for a man. It won't work if he is not committed to take the initiative for the benefit of both partners. If the woman takes the lead in the holdback method, it produces the same kind of escalating arousal in the man that occurs in the woman when the man is in the lead. The holdback method with the woman in the lead is not going to give the man the recharging of his staying power. Just the opposite. But, if a man chooses to take the lead in the holdback method, the woman can help by assisting him in taking the pauses necessary to recharge his staying power. She can refrain from egging him on too much in the sensitive early stages of tantric sex. If he is wavering, she can remind him about what they are doing in tantric sex. This requires self-discipline in the woman, because instinctively she wants the semen inside her yoni, just as instinctively he wants to release it in her. If the man is consciously trying to practice the holdback method, the woman can help. In the beginning it will be challenging for both partners, like tiptoeing through a minefield. With persistence and practice by both the man and the woman, the sexual relations can be gradually changed to something much more.

In intimate relations where the woman is present while the man is masturbating, or if she is stimulating his lingam by means other than intercourse, she can help as he cultivates his staying power through cycles of stimulation and pauses. She can also learn to perform the ejaculation blocking method on her partner in such situations, though, if it gets to that point very often, her presence may be providing more stimulation than is necessary for his training purposes. So, there a question whether having the woman present while the man is doing self-training is a good idea. Nevertheless, if it is the nature of the relations between a man and woman to be together intimately like that, then it is certainly good for the woman to know the methods the man is working with, and to help him apply them as much as possible. It is in the best interest of both partners, and yoga, that the man continue improving his staying power, whatever the sexual situation may be. If she is aware of the process, there will always be opportunities for her to help him. This could be as simple as giving him the time necessary to do self-training alone.

So, just as it is a challenging period of adjustment for the man in the beginning stages of tantric sexual relations, it can be challenging for the woman too. While he is working to build staying power in front of orgasm, she may be curbing her natural abilities to draw the semen from him. It is a transition period that both the man and woman will go through – a time of training and readjustment.

As the man gradually comes into his own as the master of his seed, things will change. This is when the woman, our divine goddess, can really shine in all her beauty and glory. Then she can fully bloom as the beautiful love-maker she is by nature. For when the man can manage his semen, lovemaking becomes an act of sexual equals, rather than the one-way flow of semen from man to woman that was the case before the transition to tantric sexual relations. Once the stage of self-sufficiency of staying power in the man is reached, then cultivation of sexual energy can proceed much more actively, creatively and blissfully.

It should be mentioned that as a man becomes proficient in using the holdback method, it becomes possible for the woman to be stimulated to *multiple orgasms*. Having multiple orgasms is a natural capability in the woman. It assures that no matter what happens, she will still be soliciting the semen from her partner, and enjoying every minute of it. Is feminine orgasm a regenerative process, a yogic process, and are multiple orgasms spiritually healthy for women? There is some loss of prana in feminine orgasm, and some loss of ability to climb to successively higher levels of divine ecstasy as a woman has multiple orgasms in tantric sex. Clearly, feminine orgasm is much less of a pranic drain than masculine orgasm is. But are multiple orgasms in the woman part of tantric sex? Perhaps many feminine orgasms will eventually add up to the same pranic loss as one masculine orgasm. Maybe it is a stage the woman must go through when she finds herself with access to unlimited orgasms through the holdback method. Then, perhaps after a period of time, she will settle into pre-orgasmic sex with her partner with his cooperation and loving help. It is in her best interest spiritually to do so, just as it is the man's best interest to stay in front of his orgasm. So the pendulum can swing back and tantric lovemaking can evolve to become a means for both partners to stay in front of their orgasm, climbing the stairway to heaven together – higher, higher, higher...

In advanced tantric sex, the woman's role can flower fully to the natural and powerful coaxing of the seed that is her gift in sexual relations. No longer does she have to be so concerned about her partner developing his staying power. He has done it already. Of course, she remains mindful of the principles of tantra, making sure they are being applied. If her partner is in principle, preserving and cultivating sexual energy, the woman can use every means she has to draw the seed out. He will know how to dance with her while preserving the semen within himself. This balance enables the two lovers to dance the night away, climbing the stairway of ecstasy in a delightful and natural fashion. It is all about lovemaking then – tantric lovemaking that leads them higher and higher as the cultivation of sexual essences goes upward within them.

Under these circumstances, the woman may find herself becoming motivated to strengthen her sexual charms with kegal exercises and other means that will enhance her abilities to stimulate her partner in tantric sexual relations. So, for the sexually active woman, enhancing her already formidable sexual capabilities may become more important as she enters into more advanced tantric sexual relations.

On the other hand, for tantric lovers who have been at it a long time, it can take another course. As progress in yoga practices and tantric sexual relations reach maturity, the lovemaking never stops inside the two partners. Then, a glance, a smile, a touch, a kiss, a hug, is all it takes to keep the divine lovemaking moving inside. Then the partners may join in tantric sex only occasionally. Or maybe never. The great Indian sage, Ramakrishna, was a married man, but it is believed he never made love physically to his wife. Instead, they worshipped each other as incarnations of the divine masculine and the divine feminine.

Whatever the style of lovemaking turns out to be in the end, advanced tantric sex is a very free state of relationship that is consistent with the highest spiritual attainment.

Before the state of advanced tantric sexual relations is achieved, there is a natural imbalance between the man and the woman that exists for the purpose of reproduction and the survival of the species. Before tantra comes in, sex is primordial, concerned only with assuring reproduction. After tantra comes in, sex becomes spiritualized to a higher state that is concerned with both reproduction, and the eternal joining of pure bliss consciousness (the seed) and divine ecstasy (the womb).

The inherent imbalance in non-tantric sexual relations is at the root of the difficulties that have existed in the relationship between men and women for thousands of years. When men feel inferior in the love act in relation to the woman they tend to try and compensate by dominating women in other ways – trying to control their huge feminine sexual power. This is one reason why women have been held down in many societies over the centuries. Men harbor a deep subconscious fear of women. Men are not fundamentally to blame for this, and neither are women. It is a phenomenon that has its roots in immature biological and neurological processes. As the processes of the nervous system evolve to a higher level of functioning, more equality in sexual relations arises, and the subconscious fears and aggressions gradually disappear. This will be one of the fringe benefits of this new age of enlightenment – a balancing of the sexual energies that flow between men and women. There will be more honor, more integrity, more respect and much more love. Women will receive much more of the deep reverence they deserve. It is happening already.

Shiva and shakti, the eastern metaphors for our masculine and feminine polarities, are neither superior nor inferior to each other. Both are equal polarities joining everywhere in the great expanse of life reaching from unmanifest pure bliss consciousness to the heights of divine ecstasy throughout creation. Through the union of these two polar energies, the birth of Oneness is occurring in us, and everywhere. When we directly experience the polarity of every atom as an ecstatic union of the omnipresent divine lovers, then we know the truth about life. We know that it is all bliss, all love, all Oneness.

The woman's role in this is on every level of existence – from the beautiful feminine being sitting in front of her man, to the dynamic force of creation constantly coaxing every atom in the cosmos outward in its ongoing existence.

What we see everywhere is the divine goddess at play, and that is the woman's role in tantra.

Learning to Relax During Arousal

The essential ingredient for success in tantric sexual practice is desire. And we don't mean only sexual desire, which most of us have plenty of. That can be used to our advantage. All desire (including sexual desire) can be transformed to high spiritual purpose, if we really want it. This is *bhakti*.

We can find within our passion that all-important desire to do what is necessary to go higher inside with our sexual energy. That means being aroused in front of orgasm for extended periods. That is when the preservation and cultivation of sexual energy occurs. That brings about the unending presence of divine ecstasy. We know from the spiritual writings of the ecstatic celibate nuns of the middle ages that even they managed to keep themselves aroused for God for months and years on end. The principle is universal.

For we ordinary mortals who have not forsaken reproductive sex, the question is, how do we stay in front of orgasm when the gods of reproduction are hurling us mercilessly toward it? By now we know the principle of preservation and cultivation of sexual energy. But how do we do a better job of turning principle into practice? How do we relax with it? There are several techniques we can apply that will reduce our tendency to race toward orgasm. One of the simplest is the count method. It has been around a long time, but perhaps not fully applied in tantric cultivation mode, which we will look at here.

We can all count, right? We can do it before orgasm, yes? How unsexy can you get? Just mention of counting is a turn off. What are we going to count? Sheep?

No. We will count strokes. "Strokes?" you say. Yes, those things that bring us to orgasm. Assume you are solo, masturbating. How many strokes does it take? 20? 50? 100? 500? You probably never counted. Who does? But now we will do some counting, at least until we can develop some discipline in front of orgasm. And the counting can help with that a lot, because it gets us used to stopping stimulation in front of orgasm. That is all it takes, you know. Just developing some familiarity with what it is like to stop stimulation in front of orgasm. It is not the end of the world. It is the beginning of a new world.

So, when we masturbate, we do some stroking until it is starting to get exciting. You know, as that train of arousal is starting to speed up and run away. Then count ten strokes and stop for about fifteen seconds. Or stop for half a minute or longer if you want to. If ten strokes are too many, use five strokes and stop. If ten is not enough, use fifteen or twenty strokes and stop. But not close to orgasm. Not right on top of orgasm. Use the count method to give yourself some room. Allow yourself to become familiar with that space in front of orgasm. That is what the count method is for. In doing so you will be cultivating sexual essences higher in your nervous system, and after a while of doing this you will feel yourself entering a realm of peaceful ecstasy. Go there. Stay there for a time. The longer you do, the more your nervous system will be transformed into a pure vehicle of spiritual experience.

The count-based stopping is a regulated version of the holdback method, used in masturbation mode in this case. Just keep doing it. If the ten-count with fifteen second rests is moving you away from arousal, then up it to fifteen strokes. If you are moving closer to orgasm with each count, then make the count a little less. The idea is to find a balance-point of arousal in front of orgasm that is erotically pleasurable and then keep doing the strokes and holdbacks using the count method over and over again. See if you can keep it up for thirty minutes. That is good holdback practice, and you will notice much energy going up, and enter into that peaceful ecstatic state mentioned above. Most importantly, you will be developing the habit of knowing how to stop stimulation in front of orgasm and being okay with it because you will find the peace and ecstasy that come up in it. That is how to get that runaway train under control. It is a new and wonderful kind of stimulation and gratification we are developing. Both women and men can use the count method in masturbation with good results.

In practice with a partner, if the man is having difficulty with the holdback method, he can count strokes also to help develop the habit of staying in front of orgasm. And, of course, he has blocking available too. The count method is the same procedure in lovemaking with a partner as alone, except there are two people instead of one, so two sexual energies are being cultivated in front of orgasm instead of one. It is more stimulating and more complicated, and requires teamwork. Whatever progress we make developing control in solo practice is directly transferable to lovemaking with a partner. Counting is a good tool for developing the habit of staying pre-orgasmic.

The count method can be used with additional stimulation, such as with a vibrator, though you may not be able to count strokes if you are using it in a more or less stationary position. In that case, just count the seconds with your inner clock, and stop the vibrator stimulation at the appointed number. You may find that you need to use a lower count to stay in front of orgasm with the vibrator because it provides more stimulation. So maybe once you have the train going you will use a five count and stop, instead of ten or more using finger strokes only. It can be done like that, and there is no problem using a vibrator or other device for stimulation in this way if you are so inclined. The main thing is knowing how to stop to preserve and cultivate sexual energy, and the count method will do that for you if you are prudent in choosing your count numbers. All of this will help make your sitting practices very enjoyable, and permeate your daily activities with increasing ecstasy.

Another way of learning to relax in front of orgasm is be still in union with a partner for long periods of time. Just being still. It may not be possible in the beginning, and we can use holdback in conjunction with the count method to assist in getting there. Interestingly, once we are able to be still in union with a partner for thirty minutes or more at a stretch, our staying power will become greatly enhanced, even while actively moving in union. The familiarity of long unions cultivates that within us.

New ways of staying in front of orgasm are the subject of constant experiment. Feel free to try your own creative methods.

As we advance in our practice, we will find an increasing ability to achieve non-genital whole-body orgasm, which will last for long periods of time within sexual relations, within our daily sitting yoga practices, and even during our normal activities during the day.

Once we have learned to relax in arousal, then arousal will become much more available to us on a full-time basis. It will become something much more than sexual arousal. It will become a full-time condition of ecstatic bliss and outpouring divine love.

The Possibilities

There is an unmistakable element we can observe as we advance in our tantric practice, and that is the phenomenon of the change that occurs in *coming*. In sex, *coming* is orgasm, both before and after the natural rise of sexual energy naturally begins to take hold as a permanent shift in our neurobiology in the spiritual-sexual equation. With rising whole-body ecstatic conductivity expanding in us, especially between our perineum-root and center brow, or *third eye*, the event of *coming* up into the third eye creeps into our life as an ongoing experience. In other words, *coming,* or *orgasm,* becomes an ongoing whole-body event that never stops, and requires no external stimulation. A mere raising of the eyes, a raising of the tongue to the palate, or a small flex at our root (anus) will keep waves of ecstasy coursing through the nervous system like a rolling sea. And that isn't all. Over time, the whole process migrates upward from the third eye to the crown as well. The delicate process of opening the crown is covered in the AYP writings.

Can *coming* be sustained like this? Can we continue to function under the influence of what could be called a constant whole-body orgasm? Is it exhausting?

In fact, this ongoing experience of *coming* is the fruition of yoga, the rise of an unending state of ecstatic bliss and outpouring divine love in the nervous system. We can continue to function in this situation, because our nervous system acclimates to it, just as it does to all other enhancements in our spiritual neurobiology that occur with long-term practice of yoga.

It is not exhausting. Just the opposite. As divine energy surges through us, it continuously regenerates every cell in our body. In this situation sex has become the source of unbounded energy, creativity and happiness in the body. There is so much divine love surging up inside that it flows out to everyone around us in the form of uplifting energy and loving service.

This is why we pay close attention to the management of sexual energy as we move along our chosen path in yoga.

Does this eliminate the need for sexual relations? It certainly makes us less obsessive about reproductive sex. That is a good thing. At the same time, this transformation turns all sex into spiritual practice. Pre-orgasmic tantric sex can offer support to the process of spiritual transformation. So, the advances that occur in our nervous system as a result of yoga make sexual activity all the more precious whenever we are inclined to engage in physical lovemaking. Sexual activity then becomes a stepping-stone to permanent ecstatic bliss.

Harnessing the power of sexual relations is not mandatory for enlightenment. But, if we know effective means for long-term pre-orgasmic cultivation, it can be a significant help.

Chapter 3 – From Erotic to Ecstatic

In tantra we often talk about erotic desire and energy transforming to ecstatic energy, moving upward through our body and refining still further to eventually merge into our blissful inner stillness to become *ecstatic bliss*. This transformation is a journey of purification and opening within our nervous system. There are numerous aspects to this journey in both the styles of practice and the symptoms of the spiritual transformation that occur within us.

We will look at some of the main aspects of the journey from the perspective of life-style, as well as the principles of practice and experiences of purification and opening that we all share in common, no matter what our life-style may be. Whether we are a celibate yogi or yogini on our meditation seat, a family person with a loving spouse and children, or someone living an alternative life-style, there is much that we all share in common on the spiritual path.

A Journey of Purification and Opening

Here we will look at various life-styles and approaches to implementing the practices of tantra.

What Celibacy and Tantric Sex Have in Common

Now we are going to touch on an often taboo subject, and tie it in with the tantra discussion. These days, it is a more taboo subject than sex. It is called *celibacy*.

Don't run screaming for the door yet. Celibacy is not going to be a suggested practice here. It will not be pooh-poohed either. We only want to understand how it fits in, because some people are naturally drawn to it. Others may be forced into it either by self-will or the will of others.

But before we get into celibacy, we should talk about the Sanskrit word *brahmacharya*, because it is the key to understanding the spiritual implications of both tantric sex and celibacy, and what they have in common. They have more in common than is generally believed.

Brahmacharya means to walk or abide in the creative force of God, which is the sexual energy in each of us. What do we mean by walking or abiding in sexual energy? Two things: First, to preserve it. And, second, to cultivate it. This is the essence of brahmacharya – to preserve and cultivate sexual energy.

We have already introduced the primary methods necessary to undertake a process of transformation in sexual relations to do just that – preserve and cultivate sexual energy. We talked about the prerequisite bhakti (desire for something more) necessary to pursue it, the various challenges involved, and the divine consequences of making the journey of tantric sexual relations. Pretty far reaching stuff.

We mentioned the tie-in between tantric sexual relations and other yoga methods, how both kinds of practices have the same aims, and how tantric sex can compliment deep meditation, spinal breathing pranayama, and our other daily yoga practices. We will discuss that further later in this chapter.

Where does celibacy fit in? It is a matter of choice, a matter of inclination, a matter of life-style. It happens. Maybe we surrender to a guru or organization and they choose it for us. Maybe we do it on our own. Maybe we are never attracted to it at all. Any of these are okay. It is up to each of us to follow our own feelings about it.

What is celibacy? Technically, it is abstention from marriage and sexual relations, including masturbation. It is de facto preservation of sexual energy, though *preservation* may not be what the celibate has in mind. There are other reasons for celibacy that are more oriented toward going away from something negative about sex (obsession, excess, injury) than going toward something positive about it (inner expansion, divine ecstasy, enlightenment).

Celibacy is the first half of brahmacharya, but not necessarily all of it, because, without prerequisite purification of the nervous system and then encouraging sexual energy to move to a higher manifestation, there is no cultivation, which is the second half of brahmacharya. This concept of celibacy being one half of brahmacharya is an important point. Without the second half of brahmacharya, celibacy can lead to stagnation and to the emergence of unbalanced, obsessive and abusive behaviors, particularly if it is an *enforced celibacy*.

So, while celibacy (preservation) is in the direction of brahmacharya, it is incomplete as a spiritual practice without activating (cultivating) sexual energy for a higher purpose. That, of course, is the purpose of tantric sex. Ironically, those who are diligent in their tantric sexual practices can have better spiritual prospects than celibates who are not diligent in their sitting yoga practices and ongoing loving service to others to cultivate sexual energy to a higher manifestation in their nervous system.

Is celibacy a better path to enlightenment than tantric sexual relations? Who can say? It depends on how motivated a practitioner is in one or the other life-style. It is the level of bhakti/desire in the practitioner that determines the outcome more than any particular approach. If bhakti is abundant, the nervous system will continue to open, one way or the other.

For either the tantric lover or the celibate, the core practices of deep meditation and spinal breathing pranayama will have the greatest influence on the degree of bhakti rising in the nervous system. It is the global purification going on daily in the nervous system that determines how much inner silence will be available. This is pure bliss consciousness, our source, our deepest divine quality rising in us. If we have that, then, whether we are inclined to be a tantric lover or a celibate, we will hunger constantly for the same destination, divine union. Whatever our chosen life-style may be, we will naturally incorporate the elements of brahmacharya – preserving and cultivating our sexual energy as we travel our inner highway to heaven.

Sexual Healing

The human race is in quite a fix when it comes to sex. We are the custodians of this great power that has been given to us by God, yet we are still to find the maturity to manage it responsibly. Hence, sex is at the heart of much of the debilitating karma (consequences of past action) we carry around with us through life after life.

Sex isn't really the problem though. It is the immaturity of our human nervous system. We are an in-between species on the evolutionary scale – in-between the animal kingdoms and the divine being kingdoms. We are a species in transition. This transition is intimately tied in with the knowledge of yoga, the knowledge of human spiritual transformation.

The primordial force of sex rules the planet for the purpose of perpetuating the many species. In the plant and animal kingdoms, it functions with impressive harmony. In the human kingdom, where mind and free will reign along with sex, it is not so harmonious.

What does all this have to do with tantric sex? Everything!

Sexually speaking, we are a race of the *walking wounded*, injured over and over again by the immature processes of interaction between the pleasure-seeking mind and sex. Our sense of self is wrapped up in it, and 99% of it is lodged beneath the surface of our conscious awareness in the so-called subconscious mind. Many of the obstructions we talk about throughout the AYP writings are related to these sexual dislocations that have occurred over the course of many lives. There are other kinds of obstructions, but the obstructions created by sexual misappropriation are a huge influence in all of us, as folks like Sigmund Freud have pointed out.

So we need healing, sexual healing. It comes with daily practice of yoga disciplines for sure. We barely have to think about sex as the housecleaning is going on, while doing the right-handed disciplines of yoga discussed in the over all AYP writings – deep meditation, spinal breathing pranayama, etc. It is a pretty luxurious approach to cleaning up all the subconscious mess. If you don't need sex, and you have right-handed practices, then you have it made.

For those of who need sex (most of us), we have the left-handed disciplines. That is a different story. Only the brave need enter here.

How do you tell your wife you are sorry for 100,000 years of abuse? Not that you are directly responsible. But someone has to say, "I'm sorry." It may as well be you. And you need the apology as much as she does. We have all been men and women over innumerable lifetimes. We all have the divine masculine and feminine inside us right now, wounded, divided, asleep, and not comfortable to come to the divine bedchamber everywhere inside us. We are as blocked and dysfunctional in our internal lovemaking as we are in our external lovemaking. The two lovemakings are parallel. If one is healthy, the other will be healthy. Everyone needs an apology for past wrongs. Millions and millions of past wrongs spawned by our rising mental power and immature nervous system. No one is to blame, but we all should take responsibility for it, and comfort each other. The hurting will end. We are growing up.

So, begin with soft touching, not for sex, but for consoling eons of hurt, for love. That is a good place to start. Dare to trust your sincere tantric lover. It takes a lot of courage. That can only happen with benign sharing, and caring for the other more than the sexual obsession we have. This is where the tantric methods come in. If a man has become the master of his seed, he will not be nearly so obsessed. He will have time to care about the goddess who loves him and who needs his unconditional love.

Most often it will seem to be she who needs the nurturing. But she is not alone in her need. Men are wounded too. They cover it up, you know. Men are not allowed to feel vulnerable in our society. Any sign of vulnerability is taken as weakness, and then the instinctive protector role of the man is compromised. So both the man and the woman need nurturing. You can count on it. Both need gentle touching. Both need to sleep with someone who has no expectations. Can you do that with your lover – sleep with them with no expectations in the gentle spoon pose? Progress in the tantric sexual methods will enable you to do this, and not after draining your vitality first. Rather, you can be together intimately with full sexual vitality, unspent sexually, not expecting anything from your lover. This is the power of tantric sex, the power to be vital with prana, without expectations, able to nurture. It is a higher functioning of the nervous system, and how we will travel beyond the immature expressions of sex.

If we work with the methods and principles, we can get on the road to *sexual healing*. What is sexual healing? First, it is not creating more injury. That happens as our behavior toward the opposite sex becomes more mature – more nurturing. Second, it is releasing the obstructions built up over ages past, and in this lifetime. It all can be let go using the right-handed and left-handed methods of tantra. Once we are underway, and it is clear to both partners what the journey is, it is a new world. Then who will not be attracted to the tantric love chamber?

So you see, there is a down to earth benefit in learning male staying power. It is the first step on a journey of healing – sexual healing. It can dramatically change the quality of a relationship in a short time. Just agreeing to work on it together will be a huge leap forward in the relationship. That is the initial payoff. The long-term payoff is even bigger – unending ecstatic bliss!

The Evolution of Spiritual Biology

The expansion of male and female sexuality upward is an evolutionary process and has different functioning at different stages along the way.

In the case of the man, when blocking is undertaken in the beginning, much of the semen goes into the bladder and this can be readily observed during urination. But this is only the beginning, at an early stage of the change in sexual functioning.

When added to intense desire for the divine, blocking produces an incentive to work toward staying in front of orgasm. As things progress, blocking will become less and less needed, like training wheels. It naturally reduces over time. In contrast to training wheels, which we throw away, blocking will always be a good measure of last resort, so we will always have it in our tool kit once it is learned and refined.

By *refined*, we are referring to more advanced stages of sexual functioning, where much if not all semen is retained without blocking, even during genital orgasm. So, when we block in this situation, not as much semen will go into the bladder. Much of it will be retained in the seminal vesicles, going upward through other routes in the body. But our goal is not to have genital orgasm without ejaculation. This is extremely difficult to attain, and aiming for it will lead to much loss of semen along the way. It does not help our spiritual evolution anyway. Long pre-orgasmic cultivation does, and this is what we want. We want to be climbing that stairway to heaven in sexual relations, not seeing how many genital orgasms we can have without ejaculating.

Now, here is the kicker. One of the routes that semen naturally takes going upward in the body is through the bladder. This does not mean we do blocking to put semen in our bladder on purpose. This will not help us, as the bladder has to rise in its higher spiritual functioning first. As it does, gradually over time, the semen goes up into the bladder automatically, with no blocking, and even without deliberate cultivation of sexual energy. See how tricky the biological change is? Advanced yogis are always having semen rising up through their body, and they always have it coming up through their bladder, though not in the quantities we find in the beginning blocking stage.

Fortunately, all this is not so tricky for us to worry about in practices, because the biology will change automatically as we do yoga practices, including tantric sex if we are in sexual relations.

So, blocking starts out pretty clunky, and refines over time. The refinement is in two areas: First, as we find ourselves increasing in ability to stay in front of orgasm, the need for blocking becomes less and less. Second, when we do block, there will be less and less to block over time because there is more control over ejaculation as our sexual functioning evolves.

There is an analogous process that goes on in a woman, though until now it has not been nearly so obvious as in a man. A woman has the equivalent of a prostate located just in front of the inside of her yoni. It is stimulated through the so-called *G-spot*. This gland releases a milky substance similar to semen during extreme arousal, and it can be ejaculated through the urethra. *Female ejaculation* has become a hot topic in recent years, a rite of passage for many women as sexual freedom is being claimed. What its role is in reproduction is hard to say. The reason it is mentioned here is because it appears that a woman has similar spiritual biology going on in the bladder that a man does. And, though it is unlikely that a woman will need to engage in blocking like a man does, the same biological components are there. Of course, the woman also has other sexual components that are part of the spiritual functioning of sex, so we can't carry the comparison too far. Viva la difference!

In both the sexes, an accelerated spiritual evolution comes with practices, traveling through many different stages along the way.

Wet Dreams and Premature Ejaculation

Wet dreams are usually the product of immature erotic sensitivities, and are a cousin of premature ejaculation. These tendencies are both mental and physical, with mind and body being closely connected.

On the mental side, if we engage in deep meditation daily we will experience inner silence coming up and we will find gradually more awareness in waking, dreaming and deep sleep states. We will *witness* them more from deep within our silent self. In time, we will know we are dreaming and be less inclined to occurrences like wet dreams.

Developing inner silence is the key from the mental point of view, and this comes from more purification deep in the nervous system, primarily through deep meditation. Some people are born with more inner purification than others, having done spiritual practices in previous lives. We can all become more pure and aware by doing them in this life.

On the physical side, we can develop more staying power in front of orgasm using the tools of tantric sexual practice. This can be done either alone or with a partner. As we develop more control of our sexual functioning this will improve the situation of both wet dreams and premature ejaculation. Of course, accomplishing this will give us rising confidence and benefit us mentally and emotionally as well.

It is just a matter of conscious development, moving beyond natural immaturity in our nervous system to natural maturity. A combination of yoga practices from the broad AYP writings and the tantric sexual methods in this book can bring many benefits.

Energy Going Up the Spine

As spiritual sensitivity rises, energy going up the spine can be experienced during urination and at other times by both men and women. Having it during urination is not a prerequisite for the rise of broad-based inner ecstatic experiences.

When the time is ripe, the energy going up the spine may be felt during other kinds of activity too, including sexual relations. The emotions can stimulate it as well – the inspirational tendency we have that can be felt operating in our spiritual anatomy. The experiences will gradually expand in our neurobiology as we continue with tantric practices.

At this stage, as the urine passes through the changing sensitivity in the urethra, it can be experienced as energy going up the spinal nerve. It is an indication of an opening occurring in our nervous system. In time, the stimulation will be there without urination, and there will be ecstatic energy all the time. It is intimately involved with the evolution of our sexual function.

Lustful Pleasures and Rushing to Orgasm

We know that lustful pleasures are intense but short-lived. As we move to a more spiritual orientation with our sex, then we are cultivating long-term changes in our nervous system.

If working with a partner in tantric sexual relations is difficult due to strong lustful habits and rush to orgasm, it might be beneficial to work alone for a while, establishing a good routine of right-handed practices – deep meditation, spinal breathing pranayama, mudras, bandhas and so on. There can be good stimulation of sexual energy for yoga in sitting practices. Solo masturbation could also be explored in tantric mode to develop a habit of staying in front of orgasm using the solo version of the holdback method. With all this, in time, the desire for lustful pleasure will lose some of its luster. That is because the inner spiritual pleasure will be coming up more and more, and it is very satisfying, not just for the moment, but ongoing day and night.

A strong libido can be an advantage in spiritual practices, assuming we can bring some discipline to our stimulative practices. That is really the key. Passion with a purpose, you know. We will know we are making progress when we can just be aroused without having to go to climax. It takes time. As we continue with tantric practices we will find ecstatic bliss trickling up and down all through us. Lustful pleasures will seem a small thing then, and will slip from consciousness during tantric sexual stimulation, and in regular daily activity as well.

Gradually, we will begin to view the opposite sex differently, and be able to engage with a partner, if we choose, without it being in a rush to orgasm mode.

Mind, Senses and Sex

The mind will go where self seems to be. It is determined by the amount of obstruction lodged in our nervous system. If our main identity is with the body, the mind will tend to indulge in that experience. With sex it can be very strong because it is the peak of externalized sensory experience. The mind being identified like this is the essence of sense attachment and lust.

The senses are not bad because of this relationship of mind with body. Making that judgment is like *shooting the messenger*. If we undertake deep meditation and other practices that purify and open the nervous system, the sense of self gradually expands inside to silent pure bliss consciousness. The senses also expand gradually inward to more enjoyable levels of ecstatic experience. Then the mind finds something more than the physical body to be fascinated with – pure bliss consciousness, which is the mind's essential nature, and also a refinement of sensory experience to levels of divine ecstasy. So, the mind is naturally drawn to an expanding reality within, and a more stable and satisfying sense of self.

It is not a matter of shutting off or excluding the mind. It is about expanding the experience of self and senses inward, and mind will go there. Indeed, the mind is a primary vehicle for cultivating that. The mind has the inherent ability to go to stillness, and this is what we capitalize on when we go systematically inward in daily deep meditation.

So, we don't want to shut off the mind. We want to expand it to embrace more and more peace and enjoyment inside. Then we expand beyond narrow attachments to external sensory experiences of the body and all that. The mind becomes a bridge between the body and the soul. The heart is opened by this process. So divine love emerges, which expands our sense of self beyond our body. Then we see our lover, and everyone, as an expression of our self. We come to live and love for the other.

All of this has a profound effect on sexual relations, producing the effect of body and soul merged as one. Everyone longs for this in sex, and in all of life. It is our natural state. We instinctively want to reclaim it. And we can.

Masturbation

Masturbation can be a boon or a bane, depending on what one does with it. For starters, it brings intimate familiarity with one's own sexual response, orgasm, etc., so the landscape becomes well known, though not with a partner, which is a higher level of stimulation. If masturbation is used for tantric training and cultivation (holdback with blocking), that is the boon. If it is used to drain vitality, that is the bane. This is also closely related to incorporating asanas, mudras, bandhas and other methods as ecstatic conductivity comes up in our nervous system. All of these are yogic methods of self-stimulation for cultivation of ecstatic energies within the body, and are commonly used by advanced yogis and yoginis, as needed. The best opportunity for doing good with yogic self-stimulation of any kind is by doing it on top of rising inner silence (pure bliss consciousness) cultivated in daily deep meditation.

Vajroli Mudra – Drawing Up the Sexual Fluids

Vajroli mudra, the drawing in of the sexual fluids, is one of those practices that occurs naturally through the connectedness of yoga as one progresses in yogic sitting practices and tantric sexual practices. This is not to say that vajroli cannot be developed as a separate practice at any time. However, it is only useful once inner silence and ecstatic conductivity have come up to be resident in our nervous system. That is when sexual energy has its greatest spiritual effect in the body. The blocking method given in this book is a *poor man's* version of vajroli, and is a lot easier to do from day one. As the nervous system purifies and opens, blocking leads naturally to full vajroli.

In forced mechanical vajroli the effort is in drawing back the sexual fluids into the bladder, which are promptly thrown out when urinating. So what really is the point in doing vajroli if there is no sublimation of the sexual fluids up through the nervous system?

Real vajroli is not primarily about retaining and/or drawing up semen during or after ejaculation, though this is what gets all the press coverage. With inner silence and ecstatic conductivity coming up in the nervous system, there is a constant release of sexual fluid at the root in both men and women, and constant absorption up into the bladder, and beyond. Then inner lovemaking never stops. The bladder has a higher function, which is processing the energy upward into the higher neurobiology. Spiritual biology happens in the GI (gastrointestinal) tract also, and is very noticeable once sexual energy is moving upward significantly – a mixing of air, food and sexual essences. It can be traced from the GI tract up the spine and into the brain, and back down into the

GI tract again through the nasal pharynx and throat in the form of a sweet nectar.

The main thing in all of this is that the flow of sexual energy ends up being drawn up constantly and automatically, and this is best stimulated by long-term practice of the full range of yoga and tantra practices.

Just as we continue to evacuate the bowels even as the spiritual biology is actively going on in the GI tract, so too do we continue to urinate even as the spiritual biology is going on in the bladder. Once the higher spiritual biology is established and stable, these functions become very strong and unshakable. Then there is not so much worry about performances like vajroli. Like with all of the mudras and bandhas, the mechanics of vajroli practice fade into the ongoing automatic functioning of our spiritual biology, and we don't give it much thought once that stage is reached. We are off into ecstatic bliss and divine love bubbling out by then. That is how we are illuminated by sexual energy coming up inside.

Undoubtedly it is better to be having a constant, steady feed of sexual essence going up into the higher biology that is little affected by urination, than to have a large infusion from a recovered ejaculation, by either blocking or mechanical vajroli, which is then mostly lost in the next urination. Hence the rationale for developing pre-orgasmic and holdback-style tantric practices which stimulate the long-term upward cultivation of sexual energy as a natural ongoing neurobiological function.

All of this applies to women also, with the mechanics being nearly the same.

Menstruation – Reducing The Monthly Purge

A full range of yoga and tantra practices will gradually expand the sexual function upward in the nervous system, including an upward shift in energy flows in the menstrual cycle, yielding a lighter flow, less discomfort, and often a large burst of spiritual energy.

Another practice to review for reducing the monthly menstrual purge, covered elsewhere in the AYP writings, is *amaroli*, which is urine therapy. Many positive health benefits can be achieved with it, including normalizing difficulties with menstruation.

Using Fantasies for Tantric Practice

Using fantasies for solo or partner practice is fine. If we use them to go higher, it is a form of spiritual practice, yes? As ecstatic conductivity gradually comes up, the fantasies will transform to a higher expression of ecstatic bliss and divine love bubbling from within. Then the process will be self-sustaining, and there will be little need to fantasize on external persons or objects. This is how it is with all chosen ideals, and gurus too. We are drawn to them by internal desire, become infatuated outside, and then take them back inside, transforming them to a divine expression of ecstatic bliss within. The last step requires good yoga practices. Then it happens like clockwork.

Do our sexual fantasies affect the ones we are fantasizing about? Perhaps in small ways – but nothing destructive. It is for a good cause. It would be different if we were getting tangled up in extramarital affairs. Then the stability of our family and future of our children would be at risk, not to mention the effects on the other person. And so too would our yoga be at risk. Daily practice does best with a stable routine in place. If our life is being flung from pillar to post, yoga practices are not so easy to sustain.

The desire to be with other women is normal for men, and no doubt women harbor hidden desires and fantasies too. Following such feelings into relationships isn't an essential part of our enlightenment process. Preservation and cultivation of sexual energy (brahmacharya) is, and that can be by solo means or in stable relationships. So we can put our hidden sexual desires to good use, just as we can put our outer expressed sexual desires to good use. Either or both can be used to take us higher. That is bhakti – transforming desires to serve our chosen spiritual ideal.

In the meantime, as we are filling up with ecstatic bliss and rising divine love all the time, our relationship with our loved ones will become full with loving service. Sex transformed to pure love!

The principles and practices of tantra can be used in any life-style. It is up to us to adopt a life-style that is compatible with our inclinations, needs, and the needs of our loved ones. If we are applying the principles of preservation and cultivation of sexual energy, the sexual aspects of the process of yoga will be served. The specifics of how the principles are applied are up to each person.

Homosexuality and Tantra

Regarding homosexuality, the principles of tantra are clearly beyond distinctions of life-style. For example, celibates have a clear path to enlightenment, as do heterosexuals. Neither is inferior to the other. The principles underlying both are the same, and the methods are similar. Brahmacharya is the key, which is preservation and cultivation of sexual energy. There is no reason why homosexuals cannot travel the road to enlightenment within the life-style they are living. No doubt many have over the centuries. Yogic sitting practices will be just the same, including those that cultivate the expansion of sexual function upward in the nervous system. The holdback method, blocking and other aspects of tantric practice can all be applied in homosexual relations.

The goal in the AYP writings is to provide principles and practices that can be used successfully in any life-style. We do not endorse any particular life-style here. Neither do we condemn any that does not willfully harm anyone.

Transforming Obsessive Sexual Indulgences

The principles of tantra do not suggest life-style preferences one way or the other, because any life-style can be used for yoga if bhakti (the habit of desire for our highest ideal) is there. So, if our desires are being turned to our highest ideal, yoga will be happening. In any life-style situation, tantric methods can be used effectively for that.

If excessive sexual activity is happening, whether it be in relations with a partner, masturbation, or an obsession with pornographic material, use the holdback and blocking methods and the experience will gradually come into a different realm, shifting to more manifestation in sitting practices. In other words, with tantric practice, over time, sex will refine to become more directly a part of the spiritual transformation process. Ultimately, that is much more fulfilling than sexual indulgence, so our tendencies will shift. Even if we do indulge in sexual pleasures later on, it will be in a way that is going higher along with our bhakti. That is the blessing of having bhakti and knowing tantric means. It is a very good combination.

Keep in mind that we go through many phases as purification and opening are occurring in us. We may feel erotic today and inclined toward excess, spiritually ecstatic tomorrow, and then back to erotic excess the day after. Over time, we gradually leave the lower inclinations behind, because the higher ones are much more fulfilling, and do indeed indicate purification and opening occurring inside. So let's take a long view of the process. If we are favoring tantric practices in whatever sexual situation we find ourselves in, we will know that we are going higher, and that it will be all right.

These writings are not for encouraging sexual indulgence, but if we have it occurring, it can be dealt with through the means of tantra. Our desire is the most important thing. If we learn to cultivate every emotion to our highest ideal we cannot miss. If we feel erotic, let us feel erotic for our God. If we feel angry or fearful, let it be for our God. If we want porno, we should want it for our God. Like that. Odd as it may seem, that guarantees positive change.

Erotic feelings will happen in yoga, because that is what our rising spiritual energy is on the biological level. Later on, rising sexual energy becomes divine ecstasy and opens us to celestial realms within.

Whenever experiences come up, no matter what they are, we just ease back to the practice we are doing. Over time, experiences will move to much higher manifestations of ecstatic bliss and divine love throughout our nervous system, and there will be less tension about the sexual aspect because it will be transformed to higher functioning in our nervous system. Even then, with divine experiences happening in and all around us, we just easily favor the practice we are doing, so we will go higher still.

Equality of the Sexes

Both sexes have equal opportunity for enlightenment. It is our destiny, equally shared.

However, there are some differences in biological mechanics. A man will lose much more life force (prana) during orgasm (ejaculation) than a woman will, while a woman will lose less in orgasm. Some say women actually gain from orgasm, yet it has been shown that multiple female orgasms will eventually lead to a depletion of life force also. These are mechanics rooted in the biology of the reproductive function. That difference is what we are speaking of. But it is not an indication of spiritual inequality. Only a difference in roles during the reproductive function.

The key to spiritual advancement from the sexual angle is not much about orgasm anyway.

Neither is it about reproductive sex, except to modify the act (if it is occurring) for spiritual purpose. It is about preservation and cultivation of sexual energy Once that is addressed via tantric methods, the differences in the biological mechanics of orgasm and life force flow between the sexes become transparent, and the opportunity for inner transformation is equal and mutually supportive. The task at hand in spiritual sexual relations is *pre-orgasmic cultivation.* In this, both sexes are on the same playing field. Reproductive sexual urges (the giving and receiving of the seed) are let go in favor of pre-orgasmic cultivation, which serves the spiritual transformation of both sexes equally. Then both sexes are involved in an inner lovemaking as much as an outer one. By transforming the love act to that for a substantial amount of the time, both sexes are engaged equally in the process of transformation going on in each person individually.

Tantric practices are in support of the broader range of yoga practices, including deep meditation, spinal breathing, etc. There is overlap between sitting practices and tantra when we get into spinal breathing and advanced asanas, mudras and bandhas, all which act on the sexual energy. Dealing with sexual energy is inevitable in yoga, as it is the primary energy of the ecstatic side of the enlightenment equation. The other side is inner silence, pure bliss consciousness, cultivated mainly in deep meditation. Together, inner silence and ecstatic conductivity go to make the union of inner polarities in the nervous system that is represented metaphorically by the union of shiva and shakti. What we end up with is unending unshakable inner silence, ecstatic bliss, and outpouring divine love. It is the same destination for both women and men.

Both men and women have energy drain from reproductive sex and orgasms. It is most often the man, because he will usually reach climax first before the woman will be spent. For the woman, *spent* would mean several more orgasms, or maybe what may seem like one very long one. That greater staying power in a woman is natural for reproduction – the purpose being for the seed to be drawn into the womb. This is why we say the woman is *superior* in the reproductive sex act, meaning she will draw the seed from the man no matter what. *Superior* is only a relative term, as applied to the ability to last a long time in the sex act for the purpose of drawing the seed in. The woman has the natural advantage in that in reproductive sex, because it is the planting of the seed. *Mother Earth* won't stop until the seed is planted. The survival of the species depends on it, yes?

Once the man has control of his seed, then he can take the lead in lengthening the sex act. That is when a woman will have much longer arousal and possible multiple orgasms, or whatever it is that happens orgasmically in that situation. But, just as it is not tantric for the man to be spent quickly, neither is it tantric for the woman to be spent orgasmically. The typical scenario for developing tantra over time is:

1. Man masters his seed and can eventually delay orgasm indefinitely.

2. Woman is then subject to longer stimulation, which can yield extended or multiple orgasms.

3. Man and woman work together to both stay in front of orgasm for long periods. That is tantric sex.

The goal is long pre-orgasmic cultivation, which means lovemaking is conducted so both stay in front of orgasm. That is the fundamental principle behind tantric sexual methods. It is also the principle behind tantric masturbation, mudras, bandhas and all methods relating to cultivation of sexual energy. So, multiple orgasms for women are not yogic, just as too many ejaculations for men are not yogic.

This does not mean that orgasm is taboo and can never be enjoyed. It only means that the more time we spend cultivating in front of orgasm, the better it is for spiritual development, in conjunction with our regular sitting yoga practices – deep meditation, spinal breathing pranayama, etc. There is no reason why a woman cannot cultivate with her lover (or alone in masturbation) for a long time pre-orgasmically, and then fully explore her multiple orgasms also. Doing so would be for the joy of knowing what one can experience, but it is not a good long-term yoga strategy, as it is energetically degenerative, just as excessive male ejaculations are. Conversely, long pre-orgasmic sexual stimulation is energetically regenerative, and desirable.

Advanced tantra practitioners may have little or no need for going to orgasm, and forego it altogether, even in lovemaking, because the spiritual ecstasy and fulfillment coming up within become so much greater. Sex becomes internally spiritualized and far exceeds genital orgasm in its scope and duration, eventually becoming a permanent feature of daily life. That permanent state of unwavering ecstatic bliss is the goal of both yogic sitting practices and tantric sexual practices. Yet, reproductive sex is never lost, and is always an option. It becomes a matter of choice rather than necessity. That is a liberation for both men and women.

Once our energy goes above the pelvis, it is no longer in the sexual realm. It is spiritual in the middle and upper body, even if it still feels sexual in the pelvic region at the same time, as it undoubtedly will during tantric sexual practices, as well as with certain physical practices used throughout sitting practices by advanced yogis and yoginis. So the energy becomes spiritually ecstatic long before reaching the crown. The whole concept and practice of sexual stimulation by any means becomes sacred in that pre-orgasmic mode. Spiritual energy is sexual energy that has been transformed to a higher purpose.

Tantra, Sitting Practices and Service

There is an experiential connection between tantric methods and sitting practices. That is the extra dimension that brahmacharya can bring us. When we say *brahmacharya*, we don't mean celibacy, of course. We mean preservation and cultivation of sexual energy, which is what holdback and long pre-orgasmic cultivation are about. It works. When we add sitting practices, then we will eventually be doing internal pre-orgasmic cultivation for the entire time of spinal breathing pranayama, deep meditation, samyama and so on. In the end, sexual cultivation and cultivation of ecstatic conductivity become one and the same and are happening all the time, even outside practices. It becomes an automatic part of our biological functioning. This is constant inner lovemaking.

As the process proceeds, the male and female components in us do not disappear. They continue to integrate within. So, while our inner attitudes and sexuality may become outwardly more balanced, we do not become androgynous in the sense of becoming non-sexual beings. Just the opposite. We become the field constant lovemaking of the feminine and masculine energies within us – a constant orgy of shakti and shiva energies. In more mundane terms, it is the blending of ecstatic conductivity and inner silence. This inner process of enlightenment has also been called the blending of euphoria and emptiness within the human being. As we progress, that is advancing all the time, and the body (human nervous system) is the field of play for this. The body is the *temple*. We'd like to use the body to take this process as far as we can go with it in this life. Later on, the body becomes a pure channel for the divine energies that are awakening within it. As we rise into enlightenment, we find ourselves with the combined qualities of unshakable inner silence, ecstatic bliss and outpouring divine love. Then all who are around us become as dear to us as our own self. Then, naturally, we'd like to stimulate the emergence of divine joy in everyone as much as we can. It is a natural evolution, which we are hastening along (fertilizing and watering) with our yoga and tantric practices. We'd all like to take full advantage of the sacred temple, our human nervous system, as long as we can. It is for ourselves and for everyone that we do it.

Moving Beyond Female Multiple Orgasms

In tantric sex, the experience of the man having good ability in holdback and the woman having multiple orgasms is an interim step on the path of tantra. It may be enjoyed as long as a couple wishes without serious spiritual detriment. But we know that our spiritual desire will eventually take us beyond that to much longer sessions in pre-orgasmic sex for both partners. Which is not to say orgasms will not happen. It is only that the neurobiology higher up will become much more enjoyable than orgasm for the woman and she will eventually want to go higher with her energy, just as the man does.

Of course all of this is predicated on a good routine of sitting practices including deep meditation, spinal breathing pranayama and so on. With steady-state inner silence and ecstatic conductivity coming up, the expansion of sexual function to become increasingly spiritual will occur naturally.

It is not a matter of the woman giving anything up. When the shift happens, she will be going to more via direct perception of that. It can happen gradually over a long period of time, or be a sudden inspiration. It is really up to (and within) her. Of course the man can help a lot with that by being open to what is happening and encouraging her toward more lasting ecstatic bliss. Women generally are less depleted by a single orgasm, though there are exceptions. Multiple female orgasms can lead to depletion similar to a single orgasm for a man.

There is much more to be found in front of orgasm than behind it for both men and women. The *something more* that pre-orgasmic tantric practice aids in cultivating is found in our 24 hour living. We go from a limited-duration peak experience of orgasm to living in a state of ecstasy throughout our daily life. It is a permanent transformation of the basic functioning of our nervous system. That rise of ecstatic conductivity, combined with the rise of inner silence via deep meditation, is a cornerstone of enlightenment.

Tantric Techniques in Sitting Practices

Tantra is very misunderstood, mainly due to an over-embracing of the sexual aspect, or an under-embracing of it.

In either case the sexual aspect of tantra can become an obsession – for or against. It is because sex is about deeply personal pleasure. We are all fascinated by deep pleasure, especially our own. It is a preoccupation, a fixation, which makes it a hazard to yoga. But without sex, there can be no higher yoga, so it has to be addressed.

What is tantra? Of course, from the first words here, we know it is everything in yoga from top to bottom, and from left to right.

If we are asking, "What is the definition of tantric sexual practice?" Then we have to say it is one word – *brahmacharya*. By that, we do not mean celibacy, though it can be that. What we mean is preservation and cultivation of sexual energy as part of the whole of yoga practices. Genital orgasm is not part of that. We go for orgasm because we need it to satisfy our reproductive urge. Genital orgasm has little to do with spiritual progress, except as it is expanded (pre-orgasmically) to unending whole-body ecstasy. The rise of whole-body ecstasy is nature's way of calling us to the spiritual realms, just as genital orgasm is her way of calling us to reproduction.

Hence, any teaching that claims to give bigger, longer, or better orgasms is not really tantric. It is only about having better sex, which is what many people are looking for. Not that there is anything wrong with that. But let's be clear about our yoga.

Are we anti-orgasm here? No. We cannot deny our humanity. We just do our best to nudge ourselves toward the divine using the best means we can find. We will slip off this way or that way every day. It doesn't matter. What matters is our continued favoring of the principles and practices that purify and open the nervous system. Life can become an easy sort of meditation, like that. Just favoring natural principles that enable our nervous system to purify and open itself. Nothing is accomplished by negative judgments. So, when we slip, we just pick up and keep going in the direction we know leads home. That is part of tantric sex too, part of the process of brahmacharya – gently favoring preservation and cultivation of sexual energy through thick and thin, without judgment.

What is the best tantric practice? In terms of consistently preserving and cultivating sexual energy, the hands-down winner is *siddhasana* – which is systematically sitting on our heel (at the perineum) or applying similar pressure by other means during our daily sitting practices. Detailed instructions for siddhasana and other methods for cultivating ecstatic conductivity in sitting practices are included in the books, *Advanced Yoga Practices – Easy Lessons for Ecstatic Living*, and also in *Asanas, Mudras and Bandhas – Awakening Ecstatic Kundalini*.

"But that isn't having sex!" you cry.

That is correct. We have discussed the methods for working toward staying in principle (preservation and cultivation) during sexual relations. But how often do we have sex every day? And for how long in front of orgasm? And how about without orgasm at all? Taken as daily spiritual practice, tantric sex is hit or miss at best. Certainly, tantric sex is wonderful, and a definite aid on the path. It can be taken to great heights by skilled partners. Even so, over the long run, it doesn't hold a candle to a steady disciplined diet of siddhasana during our regular sitting practices twice every day. This is why siddhasana wins. It is twice-daily for 30 minutes or more. It is stimulative and always pre-orgasmic, once stabilized as a regular part of our practices. Doing it simultaneously with spinal breathing pranayama and deep meditation has the powerful benefit of cultivating sexual energy while our nervous system is engaged in deep spiritual processes, so the effects of siddhasana and all concurrent practices are amplified.

If siddhasana becomes orgasmic (perhaps in the learning stage), it can also be used by a man for blocking ejaculation, simply by leaning forward on the heel. The heel then does what the fingers do in blocking at the perineum. Siddhasana is an all-purpose tantric practice.

In addition to siddhasana, there are other methods used during sitting practices for stimulating the rise and circulation of ecstatic (sexual) energy, including: mula-bandha (gentle squeezing of the anus), sambhavi mudra (gentle raising of the eyes), kechari mudra (the curling back of the tongue), and others. These methods are fully discussed in the AYP books just mentioned.

While these sitting practices are not technically classified as sexual methods, they have been mentioned to illustrate that there is much more going on in the application of tantric principles than in the use of sexual practices alone.

Does this mean everyone ought to forget about sexual relations and just sit in siddhasana every day? Of course not. Siddhasana is a foundation practice for serious yoga aspirants. Siddhasana means *perfect pose* for a reason. If siddhasana is there during spinal breathing pranayama, deep meditation and other sitting practices, the foundation for tantric practice is there, no matter what else may happen with sex. Beyond that, we do whatever comes naturally in our sex life. If we are devoted to our yoga, we will find ourselves naturally drawn to the principles of preservation and cultivation in our sexual relations. The methods given in this book (holdback, blocking, etc.) are easy to learn, and are very effective. There are more complex methods one can use. Whatever tantric practices we choose, the underlying principles of brahmacharya remain the same – preservation and cultivation of sexual energy.

In the end, what matters in yoga is the permeation of our body and surroundings with inner silence and ecstatic bliss. If we have accomplished that, then exactly how we have handled sexual energy is a moot point.

If we apply the underlying principles, utilizing multiple practices, we will get the results.

The Rise of Ecstatic Conductivity

The tendency many people have to raise the eyes and roll the tongue back during sexual activity and orgasm is a natural reflex that occurs when ecstatic energy is coursing through the body. It is *automatic yoga*. The energy moving in sex is the same energy we are cultivating in all of our practices. The fact that many (even those not doing yoga) experience these sorts of reflexes during sex is a testament to the latent ecstatic conductivity that exists in everyone. Promoting it systematically through yogic sitting practices and tantric sexual practices is not only an important part of how we move toward enlightenment, it also unravels the mystery of how sexual energy functions in us on every level.

The reflexes of the eyes and tongue are indicators of further possibilities for cultivating the experience of ongoing ecstatic conductivity in our nervous system. Such an experience does not end with orgasm. It just keeps going around the clock. The methods of yoga aim to promote this, as discussed throughout the AYP writings.

The overall process is pretty simple, really: Cultivate inner silence and ecstatic conductivity with daily deep meditation, spinal breathing pranayama and other sitting practices, augmented by tantric sexual practices in line with our preference and life-style. When blissful inner silence and ecstatic conductivity rise and meet in us, the result is an endless lovemaking on the cellular level. Then we bubble over in the ecstatic bliss and outpouring divine love that is the natural fruition of human evolution. No more struggle. Just pure joy through all circumstances in life. That is what we are, and it unfolds as we go through the process of purification and opening of our nervous system.

Once we get to that stage, a simple lifting of the eyes at any time will send us into a reverie of ecstatic bliss. All of life is divine to one who is constantly in love and in lovemaking.

Sex and Enlightenment

If our desire is strong to bring our active sex life into the realm of yoga, much can be done using the methods of tantra. It will not necessarily mean curtailing our sex life. That can go on naturally as before. It will mean developing some discipline in the form of specific techniques we can use during sex, either with a partner or alone. Then we find sex gradually becoming part of the larger picture of our overall yoga practices leading to enlightenment.

In most situations where couples are involved, it is the man who holds the keys to tantra in sexual relations, because it is he who experiences the greatest loss of prana, and it is he who usually determines the duration of the sex act. No matter how much a woman may long for tantric unions, it is the man who must first facilitate them. Then copulative sex can become spiritual practice for both the man and woman.

Once a man becomes committed to manage the loss of prana, and thereby lengthens the duration of sexual union, a new mode of lovemaking will evolve that is in the direction of purification and opening. Then sex can become a strong facilitator of the union of the masculine and feminine energies within us, leading us to permanent ecstatic bliss, outpouring divine love, which is enlightenment.

Tantric sex, while not at the heart of yoga practices, is an important skill to develop, especially if we are inclined to have sex often. It is an application of the same principles used in siddhasana and related methods, where we are cultivating sexual energy upward into our nervous system as it is gradually being purified using a full range of yoga practices.

The sexual methods of tantra provided here are to support the overall goals of a full-scope system of yoga practices such as has been presented in the over all writings of AYP, without putting any sort of draconian limits on our freedom to make love whenever we like. Applying and gradually mastering the sexual methods of tantra frees us from the negative stigmas that sometimes get attached to sex. Sex becomes another aspect of our spiritual capabilities − one of the many means we have to continually nudge our nervous system toward the higher purpose of our enlightenment. Sexual relations become an aid to our spiritual evolution rather than remaining an obstacle. At the same time, we gradually come to enjoy sex in ways we may have never imagined. Good tantra is very liberating all the way around.

Chapter 4 – The Fruition of Tantra

Where is tantra taking us? Is there a final destination? The journey itself is a destination of sorts. If we see our purification and opening moving ever forward as a result of our practices on the meditation seat and in the bedchamber with our beloved, then this is it.

Even so, we may wonder, well, where will it all end? What is the fruition of tantra? With only a little practice, we will know that it is a shift in our lovemaking and perspective from external to internal. But it is more than that. Once we have gone within with our lovemaking and merged our divine polarities, then it all comes pouring back out into our daily life, coloring every word and action. Then we have become the thing itself, and live that in our daily life – outpouring divine love.

Intimacy and Inner Lovemaking

True union is beyond thinking, feeling, clairvoyance, etc. It is beyond the idea of *the other*.

It is a paradox. The best way to find true union with another person is by finding union in ourselves. Then there is no personal agenda to get in the way. It is just divine self in one serving divine self in the other. True intimacy is 100% service to the other, without expectation of receiving anything in return.

True intimacy isn't something that can be obtained or hurdled into. It is known by letting go, by surrendering, by giving everything. But more than that – it requires a transformation in the functioning of our nervous system at the most fundamental level. This can be accomplished through yoga.

The desire for union is good. Frustration can come as we point desire outward to obtain something instead of letting go inward. Even looking into another's eyes is outward, unless we are looking from the perspective of inner silent pure bliss consciousness cultivated in deep meditation. If we use our desire as bhakti for motivation to do spiritual practices, then we will find what we are seeking, both in ourselves and in our lover.

The only true intimacy to be found is in our enlightenment. It is an internal affair in each of us – the divine union of our inner polarities. That is how we come to it. Then when we make love, we become the loving, and there is no question about someplace to get to, or hurdle to jump. It all melts away, as we become the caressing. Through practices we become it.

In yoga we don't surmount or overcome our obstacles. We dissolve them so the inherent inner light can shine through. This is the secret. Everything is changed by that one simple principle, and by the practices that stimulate the reality of it in our nervous system.

The suggestion is to redirect desire toward wanting to unfold inner truth. Then things will happen. We must be willing to act – willing to engage in daily practices. With daily practices, the experience of life will expand in indescribable ways, and so will our lovemaking, both outer and inner.

Our Cosmic Dimensions

As was mentioned early on here, tantra has often been condemned as a sexual obsession. It is a narrow view. What we find as we travel our serious path of yoga is that tantra includes all the practices we are doing, and probably a lot we are not doing. Tantra is the most all-encompassing approach to yoga, leaving no stones unturned. But where does it all lead? What is the end of tantra? What is its fruition? We have discussed the union of our inner polarities as being the end of all our yoga practice. There are many ways to describe this process – as many ways as there are personal descriptions of enlightenment and spiritual traditions in the world. No matter how described, it is the same process of human spiritual transformation. On the level of our personal experience in the body it is the union of our blissful inner silence cultivated mainly in deep meditation, with our whole-body ecstasy cultivated in spinal breathing pranayama other sitting practices, and tantric sexual methods. On the level of tantric mythological metaphors it is the union of shiva and shakti, which correspond to the direct experiences of silence and ecstasy just mentioned.

The rise of shiva, shakti and their final union everywhere within us make up the three stages of enlightenment – First, full-time inner silence (the witness). Second, full-time whole-body ecstasy (ecstatic conductivity). And third, ecstatic bliss, the joining of the divine polarities of silence and ecstasy, yielding an endless outpouring of divine love, which is *unity*. If you imagine the rise of a conscious ecstatic resonance vibrating in every atom of your body, occurring between every nucleus and its surrounding electrons, you will have an idea of the depth of the transformation. It is an unending cosmic orgasm within every cell and atom in us.

This fruition of divine transformation is recognized in a scriptural and experiential branch of tantra known as *Sri Vidya*, which means *glorious knowledge*. It is the knowledge of ecstatic bliss, expressed with mathematical precision. If this seems like a paradox, then it is surely divine, for divine truth is a paradox. If truth is experienced as wildly ecstatic, it will be heading toward spiritual precision. If it is conceived to be mathematically exact, then it will soon to be undoing us in ecstatic reverie. Nowhere is this better expressed than in *Sri Vidya's* sacred diagram called the *Sri Yantra*, sometimes called the *Sri Chakra*.

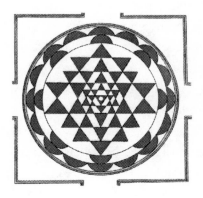

The Sri Yantra

The *Sri Yantra* depicts the ongoing sexual union of shiva (masculine white lingam bindu dot) and shakti (feminine yoni triangles) in every atom of the cosmos. The *Sri Yantra* in its entirety also represents the spinal nerve tunnel (sushumna), the nervous system, and the divine union occurring everywhere up and down inside us.

When you look at the *Sri Yantra* diagram, imagine you are looking up through the central tunnel of the spinal nerve column from the bottom, with each circle of half moons and triangles representing a layer of the seven energy centers. The outside circle of half moons represents the root. The center triangle represents the crown where the union of shiva and shakti visibly occurs in the diagram (the bindu dot inside the yoni triangle). In fact, the union is occurring in every half moon and triangle of the *Sri Yantra*, representing union in every cell and atom of the body, and the cosmos, which is contained within us and represented by the *Sri Yantra* also.

This union of polarities is behind everything that is manifest in us and the universe. We know this from modern physics – the unending electromagnetic and gravitational attractions between atomic particles and the physical objects of all sizes that make up our universe. Without the relationship of polarities, there would be nothing here but pure bliss consciousness. We human beings are both the universe and the pure bliss consciousness from which it is manifested, and we can realize our existence in both these aspects as ecstatic bliss and outpouring divine love.

We are like holograms – microcosms containing the whole of the macrocosm. This is why the effects of yoga practices are so profound. We open to and become the infinite that is within and around us. This is experiential – transcending the rigidity of intellectual theories. All we have to do is sit and meditate to get a taste of our infinite dimensions! The *Sri Yantra* is a concise way of representing what already is.

Mathematically, the *Sri Yantra* recreates the wave pattern formed by the vibration of *OM*, the sacred sound that is found humming naturally within the human nervous system as purification and opening occurs. *OM* emanates up through the medulla oblongata, the brain stem, forward through the center of the head, and out the third eye. *OM* is no small, quaint thing that happens inside us. It is *roaring devastating ecstasy* breaking loose inside us, and is synonymous with the highest stages of tantric sexual cultivation. *OM* is kundalini in full ecstatic swing. So here we find the link between *Sri Vidya*, the *Sri Yantra* and tantric sexual practices.

How is one to use the *Sri Yantra*, if at all? Some traditions use it as an object of formal meditation. In the AYP approach to practices we do not. When *OM* comes, the *Sri Yantra* will be there in us. We become the *Sri Yantra* when we naturally manifest the ecstatic vibration of *OM*, which is the sound of shakti ravishing her shiva within us. As this occurs throughout our whole body, we become the *Sri Yantra* itself. The *Sri Yantra* is a representation of our nervous system in its highest mode of spiritual reverie.

When you look at the *Sri Yantra* from time to time, just be aware that this is a representation of your rising inner spiritual dynamic, as well as the ecstatic nature of the cosmos. It is both the microcosm and the macrocosm, and so are we. It is a confirmation and a reminder of what we are consciously becoming through all of our practices. Whole-body union of ecstatic bliss is what we are cultivating ourselves toward, and this is what the *Sri Yantra* is. This is the fruition of tantra.

Unending Divine Romance

Everyone knows that sex is about hormones. There is the old joke that, "Teenagers are all hormones." Maybe that applies to many of us adults too. The more hormonal vitality we have, the greater our sexual status, and self image. When the juices are flowing we feel more alive.

It is all about prana, you know. Prana is vitality, the life force that flows inside us. It is what is behind all those hormones. Through yoga we influence our prana by influencing our body chemistry, and vise versa. We think according to a certain procedure and we become physically and mentally still inside, and inner silence expands. We become empty self-contained awareness. That is deep meditation. We breathe a certain way and the energies flowing through our body are enlivened in noticeable ways. That is pranayama. We make love a certain way, or engage in certain types of solo stimulation of sexual energy, and our inner experiences are dramatically expanded into vast inner flights of ecstatic euphoria.

Then we are both empty and euphoric at the same time. The joining of these two makes divine love – a self-fulfilling flow that needs no object. It just is.

The great kriya yogi, Lahiri Mahasaya, said, "My worship is of a very strange kind. Holy water is not required. No special utensils are necessary. Even flowers are redundant. In this worship all gods have disappeared, and emptiness has merged with euphoria."

So, ultimately, human spiritual transformation is not about external objects or rituals. It is about our inner processes – our inner silence (emptiness) and our inner ecstasy (euphoria). When these two merge, all that is left is divine love flowing out from an endless inner reservoir. It is its own source. It exists for no object, yet serves all. It is its own fulfillment, which is the common good. Divine love is hormones taken to their highest level of functioning in the human being. It is an unending divine romance.

But what of ordinary love, the kind most of us feel at some point in our life? The kind we feel in our hearts and in our loins. How do we expand from that to divine love? It is in choosing a higher manifestation of our energy, choosing a higher level of functioning of hormones, and making the journey of transformation using yogic knowledge.

When we become sexually aroused, our hormones are stimulated into high gear. We feel euphoric. We feel attracted. Attracted to what? Something. Someone. This powerful euphoric attraction needs an object. We lose our mind when this happens. The emotions take over. Only the object matters.

Love knows no reason.

What is this ordinary love? It is an extreme flow of hormones. We are drugged from within. It fills us with devotion for the object of our affection, at least for a time. At least until the hormones settle down. Then what? Then *the honeymoon is over*, and we move into a different phase of the process, a less intense one.

The difference between ordinary love and divine love is that the intensity in divine love never stops. The honeymoon never ends. It never goes away. It becomes more, and more, and more. Divine romance is like falling into an endless abyss of love. As we fall, it flows out of us to everyone around us. In divine love we become a channel between the infinite and this world.

Divine love, divine romance, is as much about sex as ordinary human romance is. Divine love is about internal sex, and it never ends. Ordinary love is about external sex, and it loses its intensity in time. Ordinary lovers cry and moan in ecstasy for a few minutes or hours. Lovers of the divine cry and moan in ecstasy for decades – for a lifetime.

If you read the poems of Rumi and St. John of the Cross, you will see that these sages had passionate relationships with the divine. Intensely romantic relationships in terms of their own *ishta*, their chosen ideal. As Lahiri Mahasaya points out, even the ideals are eventually overshadowed by the reality of the inner transformation, which is the merging of inner silence with inner ecstasy, a neurobiological process occurring inside us.

Ah, the divine romance! We have to put it in some sort of language. We describe it with metaphors, deities, and the language of our culture. After all the analysis, all the yoga, and all the tantra, when divine love bubbles up, there can only be poetry, and maybe not even that.

It's like that in tantric sexual relations also. The hormones are cultivated higher and higher. Our lover is the divine before us, inside us, enveloping us. If we have exercised our bhakti to the hilt, we know all our desire, all our passion, all our hormones are going for that high purpose in us. Nothing matters but that. Our ordinary love will be morphing to divine love in every minute. Love objects become spiritual objects, and then melt inside us. Our body, our lover, and everyone we see are expressions of God as our divine lovemaking dissolves all separations. We may seem crazy to other people when we are in this state of divine passion.

Crazy or not, if we are prudent we will keep our love going higher with sitting practices when we are not in tantric sexual relations. This we can do every day.

Then the romance never stops. It creeps into our everyday living, flowing out of us in waves of beautiful bliss. Daily sitting practices are important for this. Eventually it becomes self-sustaining. The nervous system wants to rise to this divine state. It asks us to do yoga by calling us quietly from deep inside our heart. As the nervous system opens, the divine energies take over, and there is no stopping. Then we are along for the ride.

So, if you are in love, in lovemaking, or even just contemplating love, keep something in mind. Your love has a great destiny far beyond the attachments and pleasures of the moment.

You don't have to go anywhere to find your destiny. You don't have to renounce your family, your career, or anything. You only have to realize that your desire and your passion can be pointed higher.

How?

The intention alone sets things in motion. Can you feel it moving inside you now? A quickening of devotion? A magical expectancy stirring deep inside? Favor that. Favor it as you feel your love flowing. Favor it as you join with your beloved in the bed.

Feel it as you use the methods that will cultivate the divine energies higher in your lover and yourself. Feel it as you do your daily sitting practices. Rise high in divine love.

The unending divine romance is in you.

Further Reading and Support

Yogani is an American spiritual scientist who, for more than thirty years, has been integrating ancient techniques from around the world which cultivate human spiritual transformation. The approach he has developed is non-sectarian, and open to all. In the order published, his books include:

Advanced Yoga Practices – Easy Lessons for Ecstatic Living
A large user-friendly textbook providing 240 detailed lessons on the AYP integrated system of yoga practices.

The Secrets of Wilder – A Novel
The story of young Americans discovering and utilizing actual secret practices leading to human spiritual transformation.

The AYP Enlightenment Series
Easy-to-read instruction books on yoga practices, including:

Deep Meditation – Pathway to Personal Freedom

Spinal Breathing Pranayama – Journey to Inner Space

Tantra – Discovering the Power of Pre-Orgasmic Sex

Asanas, Mudras & Bandhas – Awakening Ecstatic Kundalini
(Due out second half 2006)

Samyama – Cultivating Stillness in Action
(Due out second half 2006)

Additional *AYP Enlightenment Series* books are planned...

For up-to-date information on the writings of Yogani, and for the free *AYP Support Forums*, please visit:

www.advancedyogapractices.com

Printed in the United States
113351LV00001B/4-63/A

9 780976 465584